THE SMART WAY

An Introduction to Writing for Nurses

SECOND EDITION

Glennis Zilm
RN,BSN,BJ,MA

Cheryl Entwistle
RN,BScN,MEd

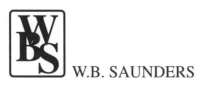

W.B. SAUNDERS

AN ELSEVIER SCIENCE IMPRINT

Toronto Philadelphia London New York St. Louis Sydney

National Library of Canada Cataloguing in Publication Data
Zilm, Glennis
The SMART way: an introduction to writing for nurses
2nd ed.
Includes index.
ISBN 0-9205-1335-2
1. Nursing—Authorship. 2. Report writing. I. Entwistle, Cheryl II. Title.
RT24.Z54 2002   808'.06661   C2001-903360-5

Acquisitions Editor: Ann Millar
Developmental Editor: Shefali Mehta
Production Editor: Gil Adamson
Production Coordinator: Kimberly Sullivan
Copy Editor: Margaret Allen
Cover and Interior Design: Rivet Art + Design
Typesetting and Assembly: Carolyn Sebestyen
Printing and Binding: Tri-Graphic Printing

Elsevier Science Canada
1 Goldthorne Ave., Toronto, ON, Canada M8Z 5S7
Phone: 1-866-896-3331
Fax: 1-866-359-9534

Printed in Canada
3 4 5 6   06 05 04 03

PREFACE

The purpose of good writing is to communicate ideas effectively — and effectively usually means as clearly and concisely as possible. Some writers forget this simple goal when they sit down to write. Others neglect this goal because they wish to impress readers with what they believe will be dramatic effects. The need for effective written communications in today's business world, including the health care system, has never been greater. Because of this, all nurses must be able to write well.

This book is intended to be a beginner's guide for nursing students who are having or believe they will have difficulties with written assignments. You probably have the ability to prepare academic papers, but you may have forgotten some of the rules you learned in high school. You may be at a different stage in the development of your writing skills and have different problems than your nursing classmates. For example, you may love to write and like to take a highly creative approach but find your instructors do not appreciate this. You may have taken several English courses already or may be taking writing courses concurrently with your nursing courses but find that some of the rules from these courses do not apply in nursing.

This small "how-to" book encourages you to write "The SMART Way." In Chapter 1, you examine the essential elements of communication — Source * Message * Audience * Route * Tone — and learn how to apply them. In Chapter 2, you learn about the writing PROCESS, a series of steps that help writers to organize content more easily and to write more quickly and effectively. Although the messages in these opening chapters may seem relatively simple, application of these skills can change your approach to writing and enable you to improve as a writer.

In Chapter 3, you review some common errors that nurses — and many other writers — make, and you learn how to avoid them. This book is not intended to replace a full-credit course in grammar and writing skills; it is intended to help high school graduates avoid errors that abound in academic and business writing. A few exercises scattered throughout the early chapters allow you to recognize problem areas in your own writing.

In Chapter 4, the focus is on finding information and on references and bibliographies. You likely learned about these topics in high school, but they are much more important in the kind of writing you are expected to do for college and university papers. Lessons on the use of references and bibliographies are taught in many first-year, elective arts courses. If you have not taken such courses, this will be an essential chapter. Your nursing and science instructors usually expect you to have sound bibliographic skills and to develop them further with every paper you write.

Chapter 5 shows you how to apply the lessons from the first four chapters to format and submit student papers. The idea is to help you prepare better written assignments.

The last chapter illustrates how you can use The SMART Way as a base for other written communications, such as letters, e-mails, memos, résumés, reports, briefs, theses, articles, and research papers.

Appendix A may be one of the most useful reference sections of this book for many nursing students. It contains a Guide to the reference style recommended in the *Publication Manual of the American Psychological Association* (American Psychological Association [APA], 2001); this is the style guide most commonly used in schools of nursing and in professional nursing journals. Most schools of nursing require their students to learn and use this method for references and bibliographies. The Guide has nursing examples, and it also gives background details to look for and illustrates the most common types of references you will use in papers, especially during first- and second-year nursing courses. This brief Guide does not replace the APA *Manual*, but it should be sufficient to help you thoroughly understand basic reference styles and learn how to use the APA *Manual* more efficiently.

Appendix B contains all the references used in this text and also provides an annotated list of books and journals about writing and writing skills for those who need more in-depth help or who want to know more about writing for their own pleasure.

You should begin by going through the first four chapters carefully, doing the exercises as you go along. If you are a mature student, you can then turn to the sections that apply to the kind of writing you will be doing and see how the principles apply.

New to this edition is a comprehensive SMART Way Web site. Students who want more exercises than are provided in the text will find additional self-help tests on the student site to help them understand the SMART principles. Also featured on the Web site are additional examples of reference citations, supplemental readings, and links to other helpful Internet sites. The site for instructors offers tips on marking papers. In both sites, there is a regularly updated section featuring answers to "Frequently Asked Questions" as well as ways for you to communicate your suggestions and comments back to us. Visit us at www.elsevier.ca/zilm.

The SMART Way principles are based on insights we gained in our respective graduate studies in communications and in education. These insights were sharpened during workshops and in teaching courses at the University of British Columbia and the University of Victoria, and especially in the introduction of distance education programs for nurses. The workshop handouts eventually became manuals on writing skills for nursing students taking distance education nursing programs at the University of Victoria and the University of British Columbia.

Throughout the years, many talented individuals have assisted in the development of the workshops, the distance education manuals, and this book. It is impossible to list them all. We owe a deep debt of gratitude to the hundreds of students who have been part of the evolution of this book. In particular, we have appreciated the help of the following colleagues: Pat Valentine, Ada Butler, and the late Jenniece Larsen, all of whom encouraged the development of the original workshops; Marilyn Willman, former director of the UBC School of Nursing; and Barbara Courtney-Young and Shelley Lietaer of the University of Victoria School of Nursing. We have also appreciated the comments and insights of the reviewers who critiqued the drafts of the first and second editions: Dale Rajacich, University of Windsor; Norma Wildeman, Wascana Institute; Reida Woodside, University of New Brunswick; Alma Funk, Red Deer College; Beth Swart, Ryerson Polytechnic University; Laureen Garteig, Malaspina University College; Sandy Madorin, University of Western Ontario; and Brenda Roseborough, Cambrian College.

We would especially like to thank the enthusiastic, supportive, persistent, and patient editors and staff at Harcourt Canada, especially Kelly Cochrane, Laura Paterson Pratt, Marcel Chiera, Sheila Barry, and Dallas Harrison for the first edition and Ann Millar, Shefali Mehta, and Gil Adamson as well as Chris Hoy and David Schellenberg at Rivet for the second edition.

Finally, we owe special thanks to Valerie and Keith Chapman and to Kerry Smith for their patience, support, understanding, and encouragement as we undertook the revisions — which, like most writings, always take more time than you anticipate.

Literally hundreds of students and health care professionals have used The SMART Way throughout the years and report that it has helped them to become better writers and communicators. We hope you, too, will find it useful in all your writing.

Author Notes

GLENNIS ZILM is a freelance writer, editor, and writing consultant working in the health care field. One of her major interests is the history of nursing, and she is a co-author, with Ethel Warbinek, of *Legacy: History of Nursing Education at the University of British Columbia, 1919–1994* (Vancouver: UBC School of Nursing/UBC Press, 1994).

A graduate of the UBC School of Nursing, she also has degrees in journalism and communications. She has combined her nursing background with journalism for more than 30 years. A former assistant editor of *The Canadian Nurse* and the former managing editor of the *B.C. Medical Journal*, she worked for five years with the Canadian Press in Edmonton and Ottawa, as well as in radio and television in Vancouver. She has been giving writing workshops to nurses and other health care professionals for 25 years.

She has been the developmental editor for three major nursing textbooks and has contributed to others. She has taught nursing and writing skills courses at the University of Victoria School of Nursing as a visiting lecturer, in both the distance education and the on-campus programs. She has been a consultant and occasional lecturer on writing skills for the University of Manitoba Faculty of Nursing and for the University of British Columbia School of Nursing.

CHERYL ENTWISTLE is director of the Outreach Nursing Program and co-ordinator of the Learning Resource Centre, University of British Columbia. A graduate of the Regina General Hospital, she holds a Bachelor of Science in Nursing (Education) from the University of Ottawa and a Master of Education from the University of British Columbia. She has been at the UBC School of Nursing since 1978 and has been instrumental in the development of a nationally known Learning Resource Centre and the launch of UBC's post-RN distance education degree program. Recently she has been involved with the development of distance education courses for the Master of Nursing degree.

CONTENTS

CHAPTER ONE

CHAPTER TWO

CHAPTER THREE

CHAPTER FOUR

CHAPTER FIVE

CHAPTER SIX

The SMART Elements of Communication

WRITTEN COMMUNICATIONS form a major part of the "glue" that helps people work together co-operatively, harmoniously, and effectively. Written communications are vital in hospitals and other health agencies, and nurses must be able to write well. In modern agencies, writing (which includes e-mail messages) is often the only practical method of communication. Most staff nurses spend 15% to 20% of their work time writing. Nurse managers spend much more than that. Furthermore, as the inter-relationships between hospitals and community-based care increase, the need for written communications will likely increase.

Because your nursing instructors know this, they want you to develop your writing skills, and almost all instructors in your academic courses base at least a portion of your mark on writing skills. Good writing style also contributes to the mark for content; the writing must be clear (i.e., well organized and well expressed, with good grammar and punctuation) so the content of the paper will be clear. Most nursing programs do not include courses on how to write. You are expected to bring with you the basic skills you learned in high school; you may even be required to pass a college-entry examination to show that your writing skills are at that level. You are also expected to improve these skills as you complete your program. Usually, you must do this mainly through your own efforts. For this reason, many nursing students often opt to take electives in academic writing or in business English.

Some nursing courses focus on ways to improve your oral communication skills, especially in one-to-one communications (e.g., nurse-to-patient or nurse-to-nurse communications). Fortunately, the same *principles* of good oral communication also work in written communication.

The first step to good writing is to understand the five basic elements that affect all communications (oral, written, musical, visual, body language, and so on). We have organized these five elements using the acronym SMART:

Source
Message
Audience
Route
Tone

Understanding these elements of communication and their interrelationships will help you to:

- recognize your strengths and work on your weaknesses;
- identify your objectives clearly and state your message explicitly;
- identify, understand, and respond to readers' needs;
- select the most appropriate method of communication (e.g., oral presentation, memo, letter, report, brief, review article, proposal, or whatever); and
- select the appropriate tone for the communication.

This breakdown of any single communication into these five basic elements may sound simple, but it really is not. $E=mc2$ sounds simple, too, but that formula represents Einstein's theory of relativity! The important thing is that you understand the basic elements of communication.

The five elements fit together as a "package deal" in any communication; you cannot isolate any one element. Similarly, once you blend flour, sweetener, liquid, and fat, you cannot remove any one of them from the mixture. Yet those four basic recipe ingredients illustrate another factor related to communication principles. Those four ingredients are the basic elements of crepes, pancakes, scones, and pound cake; whether you get crepes or cakes depends on the relative amounts of those ingredients. Furthermore, you can vary the ingredients: you can use whole wheat flour, honey, skim milk, and oil, or you can use cake flour, white sugar, cream, and butter. The outcome will reflect the knowledge you have about the ingredients, how to mix them, how to cook them, and how to present them. The same applies in writing. So let us examine those five essential elements before we start to mix them.

When you read a front-page newspaper headline that says "Student Fees to Increase," you immediately ask "Who says so?" If the source is some visiting pop star, you probably smile and treat the story somewhat lightly. If, however, the source for that comment is the president of your college or university, you begin to worry about having to pay more fees. You, the reader, are influenced by the source.

If you are leafing through a professional journal such as *Canadian Nurse* and you see a title that applies to a nursing topic you have been asked to review, you should see who wrote the article by reading the author note, usually on the first page or at the end of the article. If the author is someone who works in the area, or if the remarks indicate the authors did research on the subject, this article may have more information about nursing methods than one written by a student or a non-nurse. Articles written by students or patients may still be valid, but you must weigh in your mind the qualifications and experiences of the source because these affect the content.

This need for readers to know the qualifications of the source of any communication should affect you as a writer. You need to weigh *your* qualifications for preparing the communication. Before you begin to write, you need to ask yourself "What are my qualifications for this communication?"

You may have experiences that give you knowledge about the subject. For example, if you are asked to write a paper on care of the elderly and you have lived for several years with elderly grandparents, you have some personal knowledge about problems people face as they grow older. If the topic for a paper is early human development and you have cared for small children, you have likely observed something about developmental stages that infants go through. If you are asked to write on environmental concerns and you had a summer job as a garbage collector, you will have practical knowledge about landfill sites and recycling habits. If you have diabetes, you bring a different perspective to a paper on this topic than if you have never known anyone with the condition. So you can draw on your lived experiences.

Furthermore, once you have had several classes on a subject and have read the textbook, the instructor will expect you to have absorbed the basic concepts behind the course. If you have completed several nursing courses, you are expected to have more knowledge about anatomy, physiology, and health care needs than the average non-nurse. The latter will be true when you write papers for instructors in nursing; they soon expect a certain level of basic expertise based on all your courses. But does taking one course or reading a book make you an *expert* in the area? If you are not an expert (as will be the case when you are writing most student papers), then you may have to draw on the findings (research) of experts to bolster your statements or opinions. Where will you find the necessary expert opinions or facts — and how will you work them into your paper? To do this, you need to know how to use libraries to find information and how to use references in your papers so that your remarks are credible. There is information on using libraries and other sources of information in Chapter 4.

Sometimes you will have views of your own, even strong opinions, that should be included in your paper. In some assignments, your instructor will ask you to give your own views. However, you must still be able to substantiate them (give illustrations drawn from your experience) and expound on the reasons or rationales for your views. As well, you may need to show how your views compare with the "accepted wisdom" or traditional views in the area, and doing so may mean reading widely so that you can identify where your views agree with or differ from those of others. When you bring in supporting comments of others, you also have to judge whether the experts that you are using are accepted and whether they have done credible research.

You need to know other things about yourself as a source. As well as your knowledge of the subject, you need to know your strengths and weaknesses as a writer. Do you have good writing skills? Think about yourself as a writer. Can you identify your strengths and weaknesses? The statements in Exercise 1.1, on page 11, which are based on comments by students in our writing skills workshops, may help you to identify some strengths and weaknesses. When you finish reading this chapter, try the Self-Assessment Exercises.

Message

The second element in the SMART acronym is the message: the content of your communication, the information being conveyed. Although the message is the most important part of almost every communication, it can be affected by the other basic elements. Because of this, you need to know exactly what your message is — and to know it *before* you begin to write. This means that you have to do a lot of thinking and planning before you begin to write. You need to have worked out in your mind what it is you want to say in your paper. This thinking process is the hardest part of writing.

Sometimes the topic to be covered will be given to you by the instructor. For example, if you are asked to read and comment on an article or articles, the instructor may ask you to "compare and contrast the points raised" — or he or she may ask you to "summarize the article in your own words." These suggestions mean entirely different things — but if you do not do these in the message of your article, you will lose marks. Sometimes you are asked to choose your own topic. Before you can begin to write, however, you really must identify what you want to say. You want your message in every written communication to be clear, concise, logically presented, accurate, well researched, and appropriate. Chapter 2 contains more information on planning and organizing the message.

Audience

Just as it is important that you know and understand the source and the message, you also need to know exactly to whom a communication is directed — the audience. If you are talking to a child who is your patient, you use different words and explain your points differently than if you are talking to a physician or nursing colleague. So, when you sit down to write, you need to visualize exactly who will receive your communication. Other textbook authors talk about this person as the "receiver" or the "reader," but all experts agree that you need to think about the audience for your written communication.

Most student assignments are prepared for an audience of one person, the course instructor, so you have to consider the specific knowledge, skills, and expectations of that professor. This does not mean that you must kowtow to or play up to the teacher, just that you need to be aware of what your instructor has covered in class. For example, if you are aware that your nursing instructor supports one position and you are going to propose another view, you will need to anticipate the searching questions he or she would want answered. Do not assume, however, that your instructor knows what you mean; if you do, you may omit important pieces of the explanation. Remember, too, that instructors in psychology or law or anthropology may not be familiar with terms you use regularly in nursing courses; you may need to use a slightly different vocabulary in these courses than you would when writing for a nursing professor. Sometimes your instructor will ask you to write an assignment for a specific audience, such as a letter to the editor or an instruction guide for patients.

Frequently, instructors in nursing courses spell out clearly the points they wish you to cover in your assignments. Some state the style manual you must use or tell you the exact length of the paper. If so, you need to consider these points. Sometimes the instructor may ask you to write for specific readers. If the instructor does not specify the intended receivers, you may need to indicate in your review the audience *you* visualized. For example, you might say: "This article is excellent for patients but does not contain enough detail for nurses."

Route

The route that you select to get your message across to the audience is also a vital element to consider, and it is often affected by the first three elements.

The route can vary considerably. For example, you can choose a song, a letter, a report, a play, a television show, a brief, a pamphlet, or a novel to send your message. These routes will not be appreciated, however, if your instructor has requested a written essay of 2,000 words. There are even different kinds of written assignments (e.g., essay, review, report, article, personal journal). Most student papers fall into the general category of "essay."

Each route has its own format and therefore its own rules. For example, suppose you want to send a short written communication to a friend. Would you use flowered stationery, a business letterhead, a note card, a postcard? The "rules" vary for each different route. If it is a friendly, gossipy letter, you might like perfumed paper and purple ink — but they would not be appropriate if your friend works as a personnel officer and you are asking for an interview for a job.

You will likely learn in one of your nursing courses about the non-verbal messages you send when you are talking with someone. Non-verbal messages are conveyed by how you stand, by whether you smile as you talk, and even by what you wear (a business suit versus a party dress). You also send non-verbal clues about yourself and your written message when you choose items such as paper, cover folders, and type fonts for your assignments. If your assignment is handwritten on yellow paper with a dull pencil, then it conveys certain non-verbal messages to the audience (your instructor) — such as "This message was rushed and is not important."

The "rules" for the presentation of assignment papers at the college and university level are complicated. They are designed to make life easier for instructors who often must mark dozens, even hundreds, of papers each term. The rules are often so complex that there are whole books written about them. These books are called style manuals, and they are among the important writing tools that you should have on your desk.

Each nursing student should own a style manual. Although there are many good style manuals available, the *Publication Manual of the American Psychological Association* (APA, 2001) is most commonly used in nursing programs. Other courses, such as English or biology, may call for other style manuals to be used, such as *A Manual for Writers of Term Papers, Theses, and Dissertations*, by Kate L. Turabian (1996), or *Scientific Style and Format: The CBE Manual for Authors, Editors, and Publishers*, by the Council of Biology Editors (1994). Some colleges produce a style guide that is recommended for their students when they begin their courses. You need to find out which manual is recommended for students in your nursing department and if this manual is acceptable for courses you may take through other departments.

All style manuals focus on details concerning the presentation of a written communication, such as what kind of paper to use, how wide to make the margins, or how to list each reference. Other details concern where to place your subheadings, when to use capital letters in the title of a book, how to punctuate when there are options, how to set up a table, when to use numerals and abbreviations (e.g., "10" versus "ten"; "hrs" versus "hours"), how to present quotations, and, most important, how to cite your references.

Most nursing instructors prefer the *Publication Manual of the American Psychological Association* — or *APA Manual*, as it is commonly called — because it is widely used for nursing publications. If you are planning to buy a copy, be sure to get the latest edition; do not get a second-hand copy of an earlier edition. By the time you graduate, you will be as familiar with this book as with a dictionary. In Chapter 4, we review the main points of style you need for your early courses and describe how to use a manual.

Some instructors give detailed instructions on the style they expect you to follow. These instructions may be given on the assignment sheets for the course or in the course syllabus. These specific instructions from the instructor (your audience) override all others.

Tone

In addition to considering source, message, audience, and route, you need to consider the tone you will use as you write your message. Tone is influenced by all the other elements. It varies along a continuum from informal to formal. It also covers the emotional depth you wish to create as you write. For example, do you need to be dictatorial or coaxing? Do you wish to seem harsh and strident or pleasant and gracious? These represent variations in tone. You can be argumentative, persuasive, happy, sad, humorous, positive, negative, or sensitive, depending on the words you choose and the way you arrange them.

The poet Robert Frost knew the importance of tone. He recognized that the inflection of a voice often means more than words. If you word your sentences carefully, you can indicate inflections. An important factor in determining tone is learning to "listen with your mind's ear" as you write. If you "listen" to your sentences as you write, you will usually achieve the tone you wish to create, as in the following simple examples:

> He whispered, "Darling, I love you."
> "Darling," he growled, "I love you."
> "I love you, darling," he said.

The position of words within a sentence often helps to create emphasis and set the tone, as in the following:

Inactivity, poor nutrition, and incontinence predispose patients to skin breakdown.

Patients are predisposed to skin breakdown through inactivity, poor nutrition, and incontinence.

In the first example, listing the causes at the beginning of the sentence gives them greater impact. Depending on the purpose of the sentence within the rest of the paragraph, this positioning might be preferred. However, listing the causes at the end of the sentence gives them more emphasis and makes them more memorable, so this version may be preferred for an oral presentation.

Deciding what tone you need to use helps you to select words and phrases as you write. Consider the following:

"Hey, dude, meet my old man!"
"Joe, I'd like you to meet my husband."
"Mr. Smith, I would like to introduce my husband."
"Your Excellency, please allow me to present my spouse."

Tone creates personality in your paper. You can be bland and boring, or you can be exciting and refreshing.

Tone is affected by source, message, audience, and route, and you achieve it through your choice of words (vocabulary), as shown above. This choice includes the proper use of professional terms (e.g., "pain in the lower right quadrant of the abdomen" versus "tummyache").

Depending on the degree of formality required, you need to decide whether to use contractions (e.g., "isn't" versus "is not"). Most college papers are expected to be fairly formal in tone, so you would avoid using contractions, which are generally considered informal. Of course, if you are writing dialogue or quoting speech, you would include contractions to indicate that this portion of your paper is informal.

The use of first-person pronouns (*I/we, my/our, mine/ours*) also affects tone. In extremely formal presentations, writers refer to themselves in the third person (e.g., "Miss Smith regrets she cannot attend His Excellency's reception" versus "I am sorry that I cannot attend the reception," or "This author believes ..." rather than "I believe ...").

The use of first-person pronouns is permissible in formal writing today, although a few instructors (consider your audience) still prefer that you do not use them. For example, you should use "I" and the other first-person singular pronouns (1) when you are asked for a personal opinion or want to give one ("I think ..." or "I believe ...") or (2) when you have done the research or study and are reporting on it ("I found ..." or "In my study, ..."). When two of you have collaborated, the proper personal pronoun would be "we" (and the other plural pronouns). Usually, in your formal assignments, it is better to keep personal pronouns to a minimum and to keep yourself in the background — unless you are asked for a personal opinion.

First-person pronouns may be used in some kinds of informal writing when you want to establish links between the writer and the reader. These pronouns help to create a warm, personal tone and to establish a relationship with the reader, as in the following example:

In our hospital, we generally like to see nurses in white uniforms....

However, be sure that the informal tone is appropriate. One problem with these pronouns is that readers cannot always be quite certain who is meant. Does "we" in the sentence above refer to the writer and the reader? the hospital administration? patients? Consider the following sentence:

Nurses must take active roles in our society.

To whom does "our" refer: Canadian society? you and the instructor? Western society? nursing society? a specific association?

Finally, you also have to be careful of being *too* formal and avoiding the use of first-person pronouns altogether by referring to yourself as "the writer" or "this author." Such use can be confusing, as in this example:

These findings were reported by Baumgart (2001). This writer believes that....

Does "this writer" refer to the writer of the assignment or to Baumgart?

Even the typeface (font) you choose to use on your computer can help to set tone. Typical computer typefaces such as Garamond and Times Roman (similar to the type used for this book) are traditional but easy to read. Bold typefaces (**like this**) tend to be aggressive if used for complete sentences or paragraphs. Italic fonts (*like this*) are usually used in print to stress a word or phrase or to indicate a title. Some writers like to use an italic font in personal letters because it looks more like handwriting, but it is usually hard to read if used for a long passage. Some of the newer typefaces are fashionable but hard to read except in headlines.

Another area where you need to consider tone is in e-mail messages. This is especially true today when many of you will be taking some of your courses over the Internet and will be communicating with your instructor and other students through e-mail. The use of e-mail is, in itself, a highly "informal" way of communicating. You probably have heard that, if you use all capital letters in an e-mail message, this is referred to in computer jargon as "SHOUTING." If you use contractions (such as "I'm" instead of "I am"), sentence fragments (incomplete sentences), and the little typing devices referred to as "Smilies," you make your message even more informal. Informality probably is appropriate in messages to other students, or to friends and relatives. However, informality might not be appreciated in communications with your instructors. For example, if you are communicating with an instructor in an e-mail message about an assignment, you need to consider how he or she would like to be approached. You could open the message with either of the following:

> Hey, Mary ...
> Assignment #1 is hairy! ;-) What exactly do you want?

> Prof. Whomever
> I am experiencing great difficulty in determining exactly what kind of reading I should be doing for Assignment 1. Do you wish us to use articles from nursing research journals only; if so, how do we find these? And how many such readings would be appropriate?

Possibly a tone that falls somewhere between the two would be suitable, but example two certainly is more specific. Chapter 6 contains more on e-mail messages.

SUMMARY

The SMART elements of communication — Source * Message * Audience * Route * Tone — form a "package deal" that will help you in your writing. Most problems that occur with your assignments come back to a consideration of one (or more) of these elements. Although they interact with one another and you cannot separate them in the finished version, you do have to weigh each one carefully as you prepare your written communications. Once you get into the habit of examining your writing in the light of these five elements, you will improve your communications.

EXERCISES

This chapter concludes with three exercises designed to help you recognize your strengths and weaknesses. It also provides additional information about Source * Message * Audience * Route * Tone that will help you to resolve some of your specific problems. After you have tried the exercises, you need to go over the comments sections carefully, concentrating on areas that are challenging to you.

EXERCISE 1.1   **Self-Assessment**

All writers have "problem areas" — even professional writers. However, professional writers have learned to recognize their problems and to concentrate on overcoming them. You need to know yourself. Once you have identified your problems, you can begin to solve them. First, take a minute and write down what you think are **your** *three* most important **strengths and weaknesses** related to your writing.

Strengths   Weaknesses

_____

_____

_____

Now that you have identified what you believe are your strengths and weaknesses, have a look at the following list of 16 comments. These were typical comments made by students in our writing skills classes when they listed their strengths and weaknesses. Think about each comment carefully, and then tick if you believe it applies to you. Then also tick if you think it might be a comment routinely made by other students in your courses.

	Typical of Me	Typical of Others
1. I have difficulty expressing my thoughts.	❑	❑
2. I dislike writing and put it off until the last minute.	❑	❑
3. I like to share my views with others.	❑	❑
4. I don't know how to find information on the topic.	❑	❑
5. I like to read widely on a subject.	❑	❑
6. I like to write.	❑	❑
7. I cannot use a computer to write a paper.	❑	❑
8. I have difficulty finding time to write.	❑	❑
9. I like to write first thing in the morning (or late at night or other special time).	❑	❑
10. I have difficulty getting started when I finally do sit down to write.	❑	❑

11. I do not know the correct form that my written
communication should take.   ❏   ❏
12. I usually start working on an assignment
the night before it is due.   ❏   ❏
13. When I get started, I tend to be too wordy,
too verbose, and my paper is too long.   ❏   ❏
14. When I get started, I tend to be too blunt,
too brusque, and my paper usually is too short.   ❏   ❏
15. My writing is rambling and usually lacks a
sense of focus.   ❏   ❏
16. I have difficulty with the following: basic
grammar/spelling/punctuation.   ❏   ❏

COMMENTS ON EXERCISE 1.1 **Self-Assessment**

Just having thought out your responses in Exercise 1.1 may have been enlightening for you. When you really examine these common comments, you will notice that many are matters of organization and wise use of time rather than problems with writing — although they definitely affect a person's ability to write well! Here are the comments about some of these strengths and weaknesses.

1. In the workshops, about 65% of both student and graduate nurses indicate that they have difficulty expressing themselves. Surprisingly, most participants (up to 90% in some workshops) believe that others do not have this problem! You can take some solace in the thought that you are not alone — writing is hard work for most people.

2. Almost everyone dislikes writing and tends to put it off. Professional writers overcome this block by setting themselves deadlines and learning to stick to them. Ways to deal with this problem are addressed in the following chapters, especially Chapter 2.

3. Many people like to share their views, so this can be a real strength. Sharing your views will help you to get started with a writing project.

4. Finding information about a topic on which you must write is always a problem. Chapters 2 and 4 contain more on this. One point to start thinking about relates to your ability to use a library. Although you may

have learned how to use the library in high school, you will find that there is an entirely different approach to library use at the postsecondary level. These libraries are much larger and are organized quite differently from most high school and public libraries.

5. Another strength that you may have identified in your self-assessment is that you like to read widely on a subject; this is an important strength for those taking postsecondary courses, because most instructors hand out massive reading lists. Reading the articles and textbooks required for the course is a splendid way to gather information.

6. If you identified as one of your strengths the fact that you like to write, you are indeed a rare individual. (Even well-known novelists admit "I like being a writer — but I hate to write.") But do you only like to write about topics of your own choosing? Most of the "information writing" that you are required to do as a student or in the business world does not fall into this category. Often you must write what readers want or need to know rather than allow yourself to do "creative writing." This point is covered more fully in this chapter in the section on audience.

7. If you are a mature student, you may not know how to use a computer, but we strongly recommend that you learn as soon as possible. A computer — once you learn how to use it — makes writing and revising much easier. As well, most computer programs have tools to check grammar and spelling. It is highly unlikely that you can complete your nursing course without learning how to use a computer. Most students in your courses will be using computers to obtain information and to write their assignments, and if you do not know how to use a computer, you may find it difficult to keep up. If you do not own a computer, many colleges and universities have computer rooms (sometimes in the library or learning resource centre) where computers are available. If you are not going to learn how to use a computer, hire a typist. From this self-assessment, decide if you need a computing course.

8. About 40% of workshop participants say that finding time to write is a major problem. University and college courses do not require large amounts of time in the classroom. Much learning at the postsecondary level is self-directed; instructors expect that for every hour of classroom time a student should spend three additional hours in reading, writing, and thinking about (or discussing) course material. If finding time to write is your major problem, you may need a time management course rather than a writing course! Good writing takes time — even for

professionals. You may need to book "writing time" into your schedule. Consider doing so if you tend to leave an assignment until the night before it is due. Even if you are a superb writer, you cannot do a good job if you are rushed. There is more on this in Chapter 2.

9. One small, but important, point to consider is the time of day that you like to write. Some people like to write first thing in the morning; if this is your style, then find a quiet room at home where you can write from 6 to 8 a.m. Others like to write in the evening. This may be a problem if that is family time. You may then need to move your workspace to another area of the house or plan to spend a couple of evenings a week working in a computer room on campus.

10. Almost everyone has difficulty "getting started," although 66% of workshop participants do not see others as having this common problem.

11. A major reason why people come to writing workshops is to learn the correct format for a letter, report, article, or essay. This topic is addressed in Chapters 4 and 5.

12. If leaving an assignment until the last minute is your problem, please change your approach. College and university papers require a great deal of reading and research, and you need to start planning your paper the day you receive the assignment. Chapter 2 tells you how to deal with this major weakness.

13 & 14. In our workshops, about 60% to 70% of participants believe that their writing is "long-winded." However, only about 30% believe others have this problem. A much smaller number — about 10% — of participants believe that their writing is too blunt or too direct, or that they cannot make a letter, report, or assignment long enough.

15. About 35% of participants say a major problem is that their writing is "too rambling" or that they cannot focus the message. And about 50% often find that the writing of others rambles — even in the articles assigned as required readings — and because of that the message is not clear to them.

16. The final three items in Exercise 1.1 deal with actual writing problems (rather than with time management, for instance). You may need to think again about your skills in grammar, punctuation, and spelling. Usually, only 10% to 15% of participants at our workshops believe that they have difficulty with basic grammar and punctuation. However,

when we mark papers from first-year nursing students, we find many serious errors in grammar and punctuation. A major reason for these mistakes is that the final draft of the paper was prepared in too much of a hurry — but these findings indicate that most students do not know themselves. About 80% of students admit that they have difficulty with spelling but that they do not own or use a dictionary. A dictionary is an essential tool for any writer. Computer spell checkers help, but you should have a good dictionary on hand as well. You should also know that business leaders and college/university instructors get upset about spelling errors in material that they have to read. Instructors, even if they, too, have difficulty with spelling, often take off marks for spelling errors in student papers; the rationale is that spelling errors or typing errors (called "typos") indicate a sloppy, rushed presentation. Problems with basic grammar, punctuation, and spelling are much more common than you may believe — and can seriously affect your marks! These problems are discussed in Chapters 3 and 4 in this book. The following two exercises also will give you more information on these problems.

EXERCISE 1.2   **Punctuation**

This exercise will help you to assess your strengths and weaknesses about punctuation and offer you some new information about the use of style manuals and dictionaries. After you have completed the exercise, go over the comments section carefully.

1. The doctor of course writes the patients discharge order
2. We sent to the supply room for syringes needles and dressings for Dr Smiths special tray
3. Does the ward submit its budget by March 1st or March 31st
4. We shall never surrender was the closing line of one of Churchills best speeches
5. I want to go said Mary Will you go with me
6. Lets return to the ward said Mary so we can start the afternoon nourishments
7. The ladies coats were left in the hall but Johns coat was taken into the childrens bedroom
8. The boy said that he would be late and that we shouldnt wait for him we therefore left at five oclock
9. He wanted to go but his father said he couldnt
10. Three guests came George Smith chief of police John Jones chief librarian and Bob White assistant to the mayor

COMMENTS ON EXERCISE 1.2   **Punctuation**

The level of skill needed to punctuate these sentences is equal to that of about Grade 6. You should, therefore, achieve an almost perfect score.

1. The doctor, of course, writes the patient's discharge order.
   Note that the commas go both before and after the interjected phrase. Do not forget the apostrophe. It must go before the *s* (otherwise, the last word would have to be "orders").

2. We sent to the supply room for syringes, needles, and dressings for Dr. Smith's special tray.
   Note that the comma after "needles" is *optional*; you were not wrong if you left it out. This comma, however, is a matter of style — and many style manuals, including the APA *Manual*, recommend that you place a comma before "and" in a series of three or more items (i.e., you would write "... apples, oranges, and bananas").

3. Does the ward submit its budget by March 1st or March 31st?
   This is an easy one — you need only put in the question mark. We hope that you did not put an apostrophe in *its* (making it into *it's* or, even worse, into *its'*). This misuse of *its/it's* is one of the most serious — and most common — spelling/grammar/punctuation errors that you can make!

4. "We shall never surrender" was the closing line of one of Churchill's best speeches.
   Note that you must *not* put a comma after "surrender." That would be the same kind of error as writing this sentence: The boy, runs. Should you use single or double quotation marks around the quoted portion of the sentence? This is sometimes a matter of style, but the correct usage here is double quotation marks.

5. "I want to go," said Mary. "Will you go with me?"
   There are other ways to punctuate here if you turn this into one complete sentence. However, the capital *W* in "Will" indicates that two sentences were used here.

6. "Let's return to the ward," said Mary, "so we can start the afternoon nourishments."

Note the position of the punctuation in relation to the quotation marks. The first comma (after "ward") may be positioned outside the quotation marks (optional), so if you did this it was not incorrect. Some style manuals recommend that this comma be outside; the APA *Manual*, however, recommends that the comma be inside. The period here must be inside the quotation marks; this is not a question of style in this example. Note also that this was intended to be one sentence (differing from example 5).

7. The ladies' coats were left in the hall, but John's coat was taken into the children's bedroom.

Use of the apostrophe to indicate possession is often difficult. If you have this problem, please review the rules in a good grammar book. Note that a comma is used before "but" in this sentence to separate the two independent clauses.

8. The boy said that he would be late and that we shouldn't wait for him; we therefore left at five o'clock.

Style manuals recommend that, in formal papers, you avoid using contractions, such as "shouldn't" (for "should not") or "I'll" (for "I shall" or "I will") or "it's" (for it is). You must use them sometimes when you are reproducing speech, but otherwise you should avoid them in your written assignments. (We used the contraction in this exercise as a teaching point.)

9. He wanted to go, but his father said he couldn't.

See the note on contractions for example 8. See also the note for example 7.

10. Three guests came: George Smith, chief of police; John Jones, chief librarian; and Bob White, assistant to the mayor.

This is the best way to punctuate this sentence. The following punctuation would make the sentence difficult for readers to understand: "Three guests came: George Smith, chief of police, John Jones, chief librarian, and Bob White, assistant to the mayor." Note that the comma before "and" here is not optional because it comes at the end of the interjected description of John Jones.

EXERCISE 1.3   **Spelling**

PART A

Circle the *incorrect* spellings:

practice (verb)	practise (verb)
practice (noun)	practise (noun)
prenatal	pre-natal
paediatric	pediatric
analyze	analyse
dietitian	dietician
per cent	percent
labor	labour
focuses	focusses
program	programme

PART B

Read the following paragraph through just once, circling any spelling or typing errors:

> This paragraph contains nine spelling errors of the type you are likely to run accross in your papers. Most errors are not in words like cholelithiasis or effervescent; such words set up immmediate warning signals, and you check them in a dicionary. Ordinary wards cause much more trouble; you barly give them a pasing glance — even those that everyone usually mispells. For this reason, editors advise that the finale step in proofreding is to read the text backward.

Count the errors you circled in the paragraph. If you did not find nine on the first reading, then go through it again more slowly looking for the errors and typos.

COMMENTS ON EXERCISE 1.3   **Spelling**

PART A

In Part A, all spellings are correct *except* for "practise" (noun). The noun is always spelled "practice." This part of the self-assessment exercise was meant to alert you to the fact that there may be more than one correct way to spell a word: spelling sometimes varies according to the preferred usage within a country or even within a computer program.

For example, the generally preferred spellings in the United States, according to *Merriam-Webster's Collegiate Dictionary*, are honor, labor, harbor, color, program, analyze, criticize, percent, prenatal, postnatal, pediatric, fetus, dietitian, practice (verb *and* noun), center. In Britain, the preferred spellings of the same words, according to the *Oxford Dictionary*, are honour, labour, harbour, colour, programme, analyse, criticize, per cent (but percentage), pre-natal, post-natal, paediatric, foetus, dietitian, practise (verb), practice (noun), centre.

These are just a few of the many words that allow variations in spelling. Both dictionaries agree that the other spelling is correct and is permitted, but the one given first in the dictionary's listing represents the *preferred* spelling in that country.

Note that the spelling of "focusses" or "focussed" (where the final *s* is doubled before the added *es* or *ed* endings) is the preferred spelling in Canada, according to the *Gage Canadian Dictionary*, but not in the United States or Great Britain. According to the lexicographers who put together the *Gage Canadian Dictionary*, Canada has adopted spellings from both the Americans and the British, with a few distinctly Canadian words and spellings.

Therefore, according to the *Gage Canadian Dictionary*, the commonly accepted and preferred usage in Canada of the words above is honor, labor (but the federal Department of Labour [a proper name] uses the *u*), harbor, color, program, analyze, criticize, percent, prenatal, postnatal, pediatric, fetus, dietitian, practise (verb), practice (noun), centre.

"Dietician" is an interesting word. The spelling with the *c* is acceptable but is going out of style; "dietitian" (with the *t*) is more common, and therefore preferred, according to all three dictionaries mentioned above.

"Cigarette" is another word that is changing; "cigaret" was used until the early 1990s in news stories in newspapers such as *The Globe and Mail*. The most recent style book for *The Globe and Mail* accepts the spelling as "cigarette."

What does this mean for you, the student writer?

1. You need to be aware that there are some variations in spelling and that you need to pay attention to Source * Message * Audience * Route * Tone.

2. You need to own and use a good *college-level* dictionary (not just a cheap word book). The APA (2001) *Manual* advises that you should use *Merriam-Webster's Collegiate Dictionary*, but you (the source) can decide which dictionary you prefer for your university papers (provided you

follow point 3 below). If, however, you are writing an article for publication in a journal, determine which dictionary would likely be the one most commonly used by its editors and readers (audience and route). For example, the *American Journal of Nursing* would use *Webster's*, and the British journal *Nursing Times* would use *Oxford*.

3. You must be consistent throughout the paper in your spelling. For example, you should not use "labor" on one page and "labour" on another. (Note, however, that when you are quoting from another writer and using quotation marks, you must keep the spelling used in the original — even if that spelling is incorrect, in which case you add "[sic]"). As well, if you are using a proper noun, you must spell it correctly (e.g., the Dieticians' Office at the Well Known Medical Center).

The spell checker on a computer is generally an excellent tool because it is set to follow one dictionary. Most instructors now generally accept the spelling as dictated by your spell check — as long as you are consistent throughout the paper. Remember, however, that a spell checker often will allow both spellings, such as "online" and "on-line"; if the computer accepts both spellings as correct, then the spell checker will not indicate inconsistencies. Remember, too, that spelling is constantly changing. "E-mail" (sometimes with a capital *E*)/"email" and "online"/"on-line" are interesting examples; *Merriam-Webster's Collegiate Dictionary* (1998) gives "E-mail" and "on-line" (with the hyphen), but the APA (2001) *Manual* uses "e-mail" and "online." We suggest you choose one spelling and stick with it. (In this book, we opted for "e-mail" and "online.")

PART B

In Part B, you should have circled the following: across   immmediate dicionary   wards   barly   pasing   mispells   finale   proofreding. Two other comments on this exercise:

- "Backward" (rather than "backwards") is preferred usage in Canada (as is "toward," rather than "towards").
- A spell checker in a computer would not have picked up "wards" and "finale"; the *spellings* are correct, but in this context they are typing errors.

Some of these comments on style manuals and dictionaries may be new to you — but they are important aspects of writing at the college and university level. There is more about style manuals, particular the one most commonly used in nursing, in Chapters 3, 4, and 5.

If you are having serious problems with basic grammar, review the section on writing skills in one of the books that help adults prepare for college-level entrance examinations. A good book to help you assess your basic grammar, spelling, and punctuation is *How to Prepare for the GED High School Equivalency Examination: Canadian Edition* (see the reference list at the end of the book). Various editions are available, and you will likely find one in your local library. You probably do not need a complete course in English grammar, merely a review of what you learned in school. You need to remember that if you make simple grammar and punctuation mistakes within a paper you may receive low marks even if your content (message) is good. You are expected to have basic writing skills.

You should start building a shelf of useful references to assist you in your writing. Start with a good dictionary and an appropriate style manual; check to see which ones your school of nursing recommends. These two writing tools will be helpful in all your courses — and throughout your working life. The APA (2001) *Manual* is the style guide most commonly used these days in nursing, and most instructors in other courses accept APA style. Note, however, that style manuals may offer different "rules" than some of the grammar books — especially about punctuation.

Appendix B, "Annotated References and Bibliography," contains the references for this chapter, with notes indicating books that would be useful references for your bookshelf. The most frequently recommended book for writers is *The Elements of Style* (4th ed.), by William Strunk, Jr., and E.B. White (2000). Three other basic texts for college or university students who have difficulty with papers are *The Bare Essentials: Form A* (5th edition), by Sarah Norton and Brian Green (2001), *Harbrace Handbook for Canadians* (5th edition) by J.C. Hodges and colleagues (1999), and *Fit to Print: The Canadian Student's Guide to Essay Writing* (4th ed.), by Joanne Buckley (1998). Norton and Green (2001) contains lots of exercises that make you chuckle as you learn.

CHAPTER TWO

The Writing
PROCESS

You are probably reading this text because you want to learn how to write more easily. You want to be able to write an excellent essay in one short sitting and avoid doing several drafts. Unfortunately, as dramatist Richard Sheridan said, "Easy writing's curst hard reading." As almost every professional writer will tell you, writing is hard work. Good writers usually go through several drafts so that readers can appreciate the results. However, if you understand the *process* involved in preparing a written communication, you will save time and effort and produce a better finished paper.

In this chapter, we provide some general hints on writing that will help you throughout your professional career and describe steps in writing using the acronym PROCESS.

It is important that you have a good place to do your writing. You may do your best creative thinking in a big, soft armchair, sipping a coffee early in the morning before anyone else in the house is about. Or you may need to sit at a table in the library so that you can concentrate (and perhaps get away from noisy room-mates or children in the home). Or you may need a desk in a corner at home. Remember that going to university or college and writing papers *are* work! Give some thought to setting up a proper workplace.

You also need a personal bookshelf for reference books and the textbooks from all your courses. Add copies of all the recent professional journals that you can gather; for example, if you have a friend who is a graduate nurse, he or she may be willing to lend or give you back issues of nursing journals. You should also have some files or boxes to contain articles that you photocopy. Articles copied for one paper often provide useful information in later courses.

Computer programs can help you to improve your writing skills (and will help others, leaving you behind). You need to learn how to use them. For example, take time to learn what a spell checker will or will not do. A spell checker will not pick up typos. If you type

I was a chemistry mayor at the University of New Brunswick

the spell checker will not point out that the word intended was "major." Most new computer programs also have a grammar checker. Many students will not use it because, when they try to check a long document, the grammar checker stops at almost every phrase and queries whether it should be fixed. It may then take you hours to identify which corrections are really necessary. Use the grammar checker on small portions of your writing, especially at first. It can be a valuable tool for learning your grammar. Some grammar checkers also give you information about the "reading level" (e.g., Grade 8 or Grade 12 reading level) and about the "fog index" (e.g., multi-syllable words, passive voice, and long sentences) that makes it difficult for readers to find your point. If your computer program offers these features, learn how to use them.

One of the biggest problems for every writer is getting started. Sometimes the problem is simply procrastination; you plan to write but keep putting it off until you are "organized." So you tidy the desk, make coffee, feed the goldfish, straighten the bookshelf, mow the lawn, clean the fireplace, water the plants — and put off writing until the last possible moment (usually the evening before the paper is due to be handed in to the instructor!).

So how should you begin to write a formal paper? You break down the big job into a series of separate steps, and then you take the first one. As American humorist and noted author Mark Twain once said, "The hardest part of writing is applying the seat of the pants to the seat of the chair."

Good writers go through several logical steps, and it may be helpful for you to devote some time to each of them. Dupuis and Wilson (1982), two excellent writing teachers, recommend that you use the POWER acronym. POWER stands for Plan * Organize * Write * Evaluate * Review. Their important point is that, if you want to have POW in your message, you need to plan and organize before you begin to write. Markman, Markman, and Waddell (1994) say that there are *10 Steps in Writing the Research Paper* — and writing the first draft is step number seven! In 1971, Canadian author Pierre Berton said:

It is not generally understood that most writing takes place away from the typewriter. When you finally approach the machine, it is already the beginning of the end. Nine-tenths of your work has already been done; it just remains to put on paper what you have already created. It is the creative process that takes most of the time. (as cited in Colombo, 1974, p. 52)

We recommend that you use the writing PROCESS. Figure 2.1 shows the various rungs that you must climb as you write your papers. Most student writers try to leap onto the ladder at the third rung; they plan just to sit down and write the assignment. You will have much greater success with your assignments if you deliberately spend some time on the ground and the first two rungs. Furthermore, you should make some specific deadlines for yourself. Do this as early as possible in the course. Read through your course syllabus and note the due dates for assignments. Begin right away to think

FIGURE 2.1 **The Writing PROCESS**

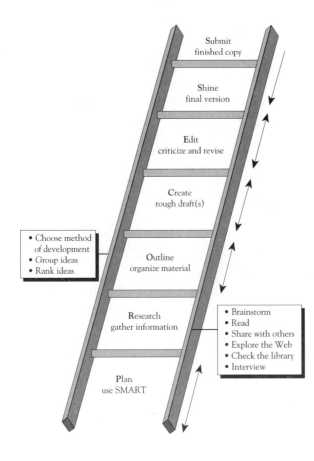

about the first assignment, and continue to think about it as you read the first lessons or attend the first lectures.

Spend the next few minutes really examining the ladder diagram. The arrow indicates that you may need to go back and forth! For example, you may plan to write on a certain topic, but when you get to the library to choose some readings, you find that nothing is available. So you need to step back and think about a new topic. Or, when you begin to organize your paper, you find that you need to go back and do further reading or thinking. An excellent idea is to note the date your assignment is due and then set a specific deadline for the first step.

Plan (Rung 1)

In many assignments, your instructor will determine the topic for you. In some, you may choose your own topic. In either case, you need to sit and think before you sit and write! You even need to determine a possible topic before you begin to gather information. If you spend a few minutes really thinking about your assignment, and sorting out in your mind the SMART elements of communication (Source * Message * Audience * Route * Tone) as they apply to the assignment, you will be much farther ahead.

If you can choose your own topic, choose it carefully. Although it is a good idea to select a topic that you (source) like, you also need to select one that fits with the other four elements. Are you really knowledgeable about the topic, or will you have to do a great deal of background reading? Is the topic one that the instructor (audience) really asked for — or just one on which you want to write? Think about your proposed topic (message) carefully. Is it too big to be covered in a paper of 10 pages or 2,000 words? If so, perhaps you should consider doing only one aspect of that topic. Is there enough information if you are asked to write a paper of 12 pages or 3,000 words? Can you get information on this topic, or are all the books on this subject likely to be out of the library already? Is this topic suitable for the type of assignment (route) you are asked to submit (book review, essay, personal journal, patient interview)? You may need to do some preliminary library research (see Chapter 4) before you can tell whether your proposed topic is feasible.

Think first of all about the audience (your instructor). Read the information about the assignment carefully. What has your instructor specifically asked for in the assignment? What has he or she told you about the topic in class? What references have been suggested in your course outline or in class as being pertinent to the topic? Think about the purpose the instructor has in mind in giving out the assignment. Is the purpose to see if you understand a point that was made in class or in some of the readings? Are you expected to answer a question in the paper? If it is the latter, is the answer to be based on reading or on personal experience? If you are to determine your own topic, ask yourself if your instructor is likely to be knowledgeable about that subject or whether you are more expert and will need to provide explanations.

This thinking/planning stage takes a bit of time, but it has two positive aspects. First, you can do it almost anywhere (riding home on the bus, waiting in the cafeteria for a friend). Second, it gets you started. And, if you like to be creative, it can be a highly stimulating time.

RESEARCH (RUNG 2)

After thinking about the five SMART elements, as in Chapter 1, you will probably need to do some preliminary research before you can decide definitely on your topic and work out the plan for the next steps. For your first nursing assignments, usually this means doing some extra reading about what experts have said about the topic. In most courses, your instructors will give you lists of readings, and some of them likely apply to your topic. However, you should do additional research in a good library.

Once you have determined the topic, you can start to gather the information. You should also talk to others about the topic. Chatting informally over coffee with fellow students or visiting the chat rooms or forums set up on the Web for your course might give you some ideas. Remember, you do not have to use these ideas if they do not fit with what *you*, the source, want to say. You might discuss the subject over dinner with non-nursing friends or family; you might be surprised to find that family members can suggest some good ideas! As well, you can browse on the Internet and in the library and begin to set up a working bibliography (as described in Chapter 4).

OUTLINE (RUNG 3)

The next step on the ladder is to organize your information into an intelligent plan for communicating it in your paper. You may find it helpful to brainstorm. Sit down with a piece of paper and jot down (briefly, using only one or two words) all the ideas that you want to develop in the assignment. You might prefer to do this as a list, but others might like to do it as a "map" in which they put the central idea in the centre of a page and then group other ideas around it. When a subidea sparks other ideas, you group them around the subidea. Some instructors refer to this idea as "clustering."

For example, suppose your instructor has asked you to write a short assignment describing what you believe the image of a professional nurse is like. This is part of the topic of professionalism, which was discussed in one of your lectures. You have been assigned some readings on the topic, and these should get you started. We have given the beginnings of a "map" on this topic in Figure 2.2. Not all of you will want to draw a map like this one. You may prefer to make a list of your ideas.

Once you have come up with all the ideas that you want to put into your assignment, you need to organize them into some sort of order — you need an

FIGURE 2.2   **Brainstorming Map**

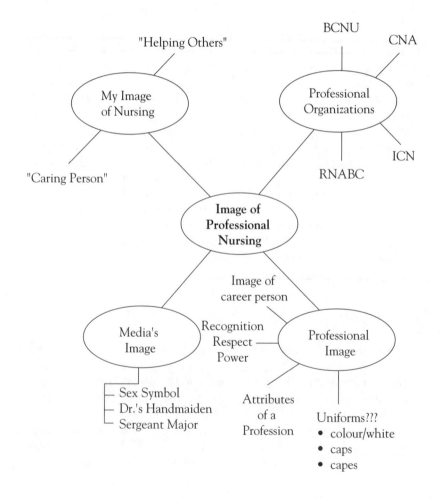

outline. You should remember the outline, because you learned about it in elementary school when you were first learning how to write essays. See Box 2.1.

You will remember that your elementary schoolteachers urged you to organize your papers into *three* main parts. This is still a good idea, although it will not work for all topics. Some topics need two parts, while some need four or more parts. The rationale behind this division into main parts, however, is that readers will be able to follow your thoughts. Keeping the main divisions to a manageable number (such as three) helps readers to grasp your ideas readily and to remember them easily. You may cover more than three ideas within a paper, but some of them will be organized as subparts of one of the three main ideas.

You also help your readers to understand your message by telling them in the introduction just what you are going to cover in the main part of the paper. And in the concluding section, you sum up your ideas briefly to remind the reader what was covered. In the journalistic world, this organizational pattern is summed up this way:

- Tell them what you are going to tell them.
- Tell them.
- Tell them what you have told them.

This framework may sound rather simplistic, but you can still be creative within it. Remember that an assignment is not a mystery novel in which you save your point until the end of the book. Making your point clearly in the

BOX 2.1 Outline

OUTLINE
I. Introduction
II. Body
   A. First main idea
      1. Subidea to main idea
      2. Subidea to main idea
         a. sub-subidea
         b. sub-subidea
   B. Second main idea
     (and subideas organized as in A)
   C. Third main idea
     (and subideas organized as in A)
III. Conclusion

introduction will certainly help your instructor to understand what you are doing with your paper — and will likely pay off in marks!

Students who have major problems with written communications have failed to spend time on the three basic first steps of the ladder. Furthermore, these early steps are usually the fun part of writing. They represent the time when you can let your imagination flow.

You may want to finish the outline stage by jotting down several ideas for a title; doing so helps you to define your idea. Let your mind go; be creative. Try to summarize the main idea in one or two sentences or in those famous "25 words or less." If you start early enough, you can take a few minutes a day for several days in this phase. And you can do it anywhere, such as while driving to work or washing the car. Just be sure that you jot down the ideas for later use.

During the brainstorming stage, jot down as many ideas as possible — you can never have too many ideas during brainstorming. In the outlining stage, however, you need to consider the length of the final paper. Almost all instructors specify length. Some instructors take off marks if a student writes a paper that is longer than specified. If at this point — *before* you begin to write — you consider the overall length, you can focus on the most important ideas and group the less important ideas so that you cover the greatest amount of information without putting too much emphasis on one point. You can decide to omit some details, or you can select one example to stand for several others. If you are conscious of length right from the beginning, likely you will not have to spend hours later trying to shorten a lengthy draft. As well, you will be less likely to ramble once you begin to write.

CREATE (RUNG 4)

If you spend time on the three early rungs, then you should be able to write your first drafts for papers much more quickly than you have in the past. However, you should still plan on having to make at least one rough draft. Most professional writers say they need at least three. This does not necessarily mean that you copy out your draft word for word each time. What you do is create a "working draft" that you can go over several times. If you work on a computer, this is easy. You can alter your original draft quickly.

Even if you have not yet joined the computer generation, you can still create a working draft that is easy to alter. Write or type your first draft using only every second or third line (i.e., double- or triple-spaced), and use WIDE margins. Many student nurses simply will not do this; they seem determined not to "waste" paper and thus cover every page from corner to corner, using every possible bit of space. Overcome this tendency! If you double-space your writing, then you can go over the paper a second time (and third and fourth, if necessary) and simply add or delete words and phrases. You can write in the margins if you leave them wide enough. You can insert an asterisk (*) and turn the page over and add a sentence or two. You can cross out words and substitute better or clearer words above them. You can correct your spelling and grammar without having to crowd your words. You, or your typist, will be able to read your draft more easily.

Ideally, you should create the first working copy quickly. A first draft should be creative and should flow. In early drafts, you concentrate on developing the main body of the message. From your brainstorming and outlining sessions, you know what the main points of your message are, and you will have organized them to make your message clear and strong, keeping your audience in mind. You should be able to pick up words and phrases directly from your brainstorming page and outline and incorporate them into the first draft.

You may still find it hard to start writing at this point. The best way is simply to begin. Put some sentences down on your paper or on the screen of your computer. Simply by writing half a page or more, you get started. You may eventually scrap it, but you have started. This approach is called "free writing."

Some instructors, especially during first-year courses, often try to help students overcome a writing block by giving short assignments designed to help you improve both your writing and your thinking skills. These assignments often are described as "writing-to-learn" projects and are designed to help student nurses acquire and interpret (for themselves as well as for others) the complex knowledge base needed in nursing. Such projects help students to clarify theoretical points or to reflect on ways that personal experiences ("lived experiences") can be applied; they are intended to help students develop conceptual approaches and thinking patterns that will be helpful in practice settings.

Such projects often involve "free writing" and "quick writing." Free writing often is assigned at the beginning of a class. Students spend about five minutes writing about their feelings (e.g., feelings after the first visit to a hospital ward or after the death of a patient), or about concerns or issues involving the students (e.g., thoughts about a proposed student strike to protest a fee hike), or about a previous class or assignment (e.g., summaries of articles assigned as reading). For most of these "quick-write" assignments, instructors are concerned only with your ability to identify the main points or concepts (message) and are not as interested in grammar, spelling, punctuation, sentence and paragraph construction, and presentation (matters of route). However, these instructors may also use these writing-to-learn assignments to provide feedback about writing skills; because the papers usually are short, an instructor takes time to identify writing skill problems as well as to assess conceptualization skills.

Many instructors ask students to keep a daily (or weekly) log or journal in which they describe their feelings, summarize their classroom or clinical learning, or raise issues for discussion in class. This is often referred to as "journalling." These assignments are usually informal writings that you keep for your own personal use — although in this case you allow your instructor, and maybe your classmates, to share your thoughts. The principle behind these assignments is to get you to use words to capture ideas. And because you are choosing words to express your own thoughts, feelings, opinions, impressions, beliefs, emotions, or concerns, you do it without having to turn to the writings of others. This gives you practice with thinking in words and putting these on paper so others can see your views and understand them. Such assignments help you to understand more about what you think and feel. For, as the English poet George Gordon, Lord Byron (as cited in Colombo, 1974, p. 91) wrote,

> ... words are things, and a small drop of ink,
> Falling like dew, upon a thought, produces
> That which makes thousands, perhaps millions think.

You often learn from these small exercises that you really do have good writing skills, and that you do have thoughts that are meaningful and worth sharing. Some instructors ask students to write poetry as one way of getting in touch with their feelings through the experience of capturing these in words — and some of these poems are real gems.

Usually your instructor will tell you how he or she wishes the journal or the quick-writes to be set up (the rules of the route), such as handwritten in a small scribbler or written double-spaced on lined paper with one wide margin for feedback. For these writing-to-learn projects, you still need to think SMART and to go through the steps that make up the writing process — even though you must do it more quickly than with a longer paper.

You can practise free writing or quick writing on your own. Writing things down helps you to clarify theoretical points or reflect on ways that personal experiences (sometimes called "lived experiences") can be applied. Such practice helps you to develop conceptual approaches and thinking patterns that will also be helpful in practice settings.

Once you are caught up in the flow of the writing, your thoughts will become more organized. Many writers like to complete the body of the paper first and then turn to the introduction and conclusion. Other writers like to write the introduction first because it helps them to clarify exactly what they want to say and the order in which to say it. Either way, you want to keep the introductory and concluding sections short, especially during the first draft. You can come back to them during the next steps when you edit and revise.

Writing the first draft is not the time to worry about spelling or grammar; you can fix these later. Look quickly to see that you have the references on hand as you mention them in the draft, but do not worry about getting them copied down in detail; leave this for later.

At this point, you should be trying to put the message into your own words, showing that you truly understand what it is. Be creative, remembering that this is merely the *beginning* of the paper; knowing that this version does not have to be perfect helps you to let your ideas flow. Visualize your instructor reading it. See your paper as a kind of long, informative letter with a specific message from you. Focus on getting your whole message across.

Once you have your first draft finished, try to leave it as is and take a break. If you can leave it overnight and do the editing and revising the next day, you will likely be able to read the paper over and easily spot areas that need to be worked on further. If you are organized enough to be preparing the paper several days in advance, then you will even have time to do a bit more research if necessary.

When you come back to your first draft, continue at first to concentrate on the message rather than on details of spelling and grammar. Ask yourself if you got the main point across clearly so that any reader could understand it. Are the subordinate points obvious so that the reader can follow them clearly? You may want to add more in one section, elaborate some point, or give an example to make your point clearly. If you work on a computer, these revisions are easy. If not, you can get the scissors and cut and paste or tape. All good writers have revised their drafts, from Charles Dickens to Ernest Hemingway to Stephen King.

Keep considering the length as you work. If you work on a computer, you will find it easy to work out the length. If you are still writing your papers by hand, count the number of words on a typical page and estimate the number of pages that you will need for the finished copy. Keep this number in mind for future papers. (If you must do a count, include all the little words such as "a," "the," and "I.")

Eventually, you will achieve a copy that contains the message you are satisfied with — or, more likely, you will run short of time! Either way, you need to go over the draft version once more.

EDIT (RUNG 5)

During the final review of the draft, you stop creating the message and start to concentrate on critiquing and improving the writing. Now is the time to look at vocabulary, grammar, punctuation, and spelling. This is the time to consider the tone of the essay. Is it too formal? Have you used appropriate language for a college-level paper? Have you used the appropriate vocabulary for your level of nursing ("abdomen" rather than "tummy"; "intestine" rather than "gut")? Have you borrowed jargon from the readings without really understanding it? Are your words too pretentious? A general rule is that clear, simple, appropriate words convey your message the best. Use your critical faculties. Stop looking at what you want to say and concentrate on saying it well and clearly.

When you begin to revise, concentrate especially on good, clear writing in the introductory and concluding sections of the paper. They are vital because they make the most impact on readers. You want to start with some strong, clearly stated, and, if possible, memorable sentences. And you want to end your message by clearly reviewing what you tried to achieve in the body of the paper. The words of your final paragraph will leave a lasting impression on your instructor as he or she works out your mark. So consider these sections carefully. Many great authors suggest that you spend as much time on the first and the last paragraphs as you do on the rest of the paper!

In the editing of your paper, you must concentrate on the "flow" of ideas and be certain that these are obvious to the reader (audience). Nursing instructors frequently stress to us the importance of "flow" and tell us that students fail to understand this point. You may find that some instructors will write this onto your paper as they mark it. "Flow" refers to the logical streaming of ideas throughout the paper from beginning to end. Often you will have good ideas, but if you do not link them in a clear, logical order, readers (audience) will find it difficult to understand the rationale and to follow the reasoning in your argument.

Clear flow is helped by little "road signs" that you put into your paper, such as "First, I want to ...." and then, later in the paper, you write another marker, such as "Second, I propose to ...." Other such markers, which often come at the beginning of new paragraphs, are:

"Next, ..."
"On the other hand, ..." (Just be careful you do not have more than two hands!)
"In contrast to the idea discussed in the paragraphs above, ..."

These road markers, often described in writing textbooks as "transitions" or as "linking words or phrases," help the reader to follow your argument.

A useful hint at this stage is to read the paper out loud to yourself, listening to the words and grammar rather than to the message. Does the sentence sound right, or can it be misinterpreted? Consider these newspaper headlines that slipped by editors:

"Drunken Drivers Paid $1,000 Last Week"
"Local High School Dropouts Cut in Half"
"Miners Refuse to Work after Death"

Watch out for sentences that are too long to read comfortably. Do you get lost halfway through a sentence? Do you fail to understand what a pronoun refers to? If you have trouble with it, think how difficult it will be for your instructor or other readers.

If the draft is not too messy, get someone else to read it — but either provide a photocopy or tell the person not to write on your version. (Give him or her some Post-it notes.) Try to find someone who is helpful but not overly critical; all writers are vulnerable when they give a draft to someone to review! The person need not be an expert on the content, but pick someone who can learn from reading your paper — and he or she will only learn from it if it is clearly written. You want a friend who will offer some praise and positive feedback as well as some useful critical comments. Remember, too, that you do not have to accept and use all the criticisms. Chapter 3 gives more detail on these and other points to look for when you are editing the final draft.

SHINE (RUNG 6)

Now is the time for you to "shine" or polish your work. As you print out or type up the final copy — or just before you send it to the typist — look at the general format of the paper, such as headings, spacing, table of contents, size of type, and so on. Also consider your quotations, citations, and references. These are all points related to the route — and, for first-year student papers, they are covered in Chapters 4 and 5. If you are in a more senior year, you probably need a style manual that spells out the rules of the route in more detail. Or, if you are looking at the rules for other presentations (business letters, résumés, business reports), you should review Chapter 6.

You need to turn in a final version that is clean and easy to read. Just as you would not appear for a job interview in dirty, ragged gardening clothes, so your paper must appear on the instructor's desk in a suitable form. Unless you have made other arrangements with the instructor, you should turn in a typed or printed hard copy. A few instructors will allow you to turn in a handwritten version, but, if so, it must be legible and follow the general rules for papers. Some instructors may also allow you to submit your paper electronically — but there still may be some difficulties with such submissions. See Chapter 5 for more about this.

Some instructors like to receive assignments in folders or envelopes. If so, they will usually specify this in the assignment handouts. Sometimes the route specified in the assignment dictates what you use (e.g., a nursing chart page). Most often, however, you should simply turn in an assignment paper as advised in the style sheet or manual recommended for use by your department. Most style sheets and manuals suggest that you gather the pages together with a paper clip; a few recommend using a staple in the top left corner. These rules are meant to make it easier for the instructor to carry, read, and mark up your assignment.

Instructors often want or need a few extra things in a student paper that may not be specified in a style manual. For example, a distance education student may decide to attach a cover letter (probably only one page) to the paper. Cover letters allow you to give additional details that may not be appropriate in a formal paper. For example, the letter might explain why the paper is late (or early, as the case may be). Or you may need to indicate that you are going to be away temporarily and need to have the paper returned to some other address. If you use a cover letter, it should be set up properly as a business letter — although it need not be typed.

As a final step, you should read over the hard copy before you turn it in. You may find a few typing errors (e.g., "works" instead of "words") that slipped by previous proofreading or were not picked up on the spell checker. Or you may find a place where there was a small breakdown in the computer codes that caused minor errors or typos in a few words or lines. You can correct these mistakes neatly in ink on the final copy or use a clean eraser or a bit of "white out" solution to tidy up the page. You will not lose marks if you make the corrections clearly and neatly, but you probably will if you simply leave the typo or the error.

SUBMIT (RUNG 7)

The final step in the writing process is to submit the paper on time. Some instructors deduct marks for a paper that is late. One reason for doing so is that if other students manage to meet the deadline you have an unfair advantage. Check the policies of your school. On the other hand, most instructors will grant you an extension when there is a legitimate reason. Ask!

SUMMARY

In this chapter, we have provided a number of ideas that are useful to writers, including some general hints, and have described a specific writing process that has proven useful for a generation of student nurses. If you look back, you will see that the initial letters for each of the steps spell out PROCESS.

Plan
Research
Outline
Create
Edit
Shine
Submit

This acronym will help you to understand that good writing has several steps — and, if you want to write like a pro, the most important steps occur before you sit down to write.

EXERCISES

We have included self-assessment exercises on mapping and outlining to give you some practice using these two parts of the process.

EXERCISE 2.1   Brainstorming

Try a five-minute brainstorming session and make a map of some topic for a 10-page college-level paper. You might try "Making a Hospital Bed," or "Pros and Cons of Wearing a Uniform in Nursing," or any other topic.

COMMENTS ON EXERCISE 2.1   Brainstorming

Refer to the map in Figure 2.2 for ideas about mapping. Following, however, are some points to keep in mind.

Even in this exercise, you need to consider all the SMART elements. Suppose you have decided to tackle "Pros and Cons of Wearing a Uniform in Nursing." You (source) may have some definite opinions on this topic. The first map likely will reflect some of the questions that arise in your own mind, such as "Should nurses wear a uniform?" But as you think about this for a few minutes, other questions may arise about the message, such as:

- "Why did nurses wear standard uniforms that represented their schools of nursing? Why did they wear caps? Why did they stop wearing standard uniforms — and when?" Perhaps you could even make a big circle around these points and list them as "History of Uniforms in Nursing."

- "Do other professionals wear uniforms?"
- "Does wearing a uniform take away your individuality?"
- "Does a uniform contribute to (or take away from) a professional image?"
- "Should uniforms be white or colored — and why?"
- "What do patients think about nurses' uniforms?"
- "Should the uniform be typical of the hospital in which you are working?"
- "Should the uniform reflect the department, such as the operating room or emergency department?"

You, and various people you may talk to, including other students, graduate nurses, and patients, may raise other points. But you also need to think about the course for which this paper is required: Did you discuss "the image of nursing" or "professionalism" in your classes — and were uniforms mentioned in the discussion? Did any of your assigned readings raise the topic of uniforms? Are uniforms mentioned in your textbook readings? Will your instructor (audience) expect you to refer to some of these points?

In the early mapping, you should write down as many ideas as you can think of — whether or not these are pros or cons. Then, if you have strong opinions one way or the other, you may want to make your paper reflect these and come to a conclusion that nurses should (or should not) wear a standard uniform on the wards. Thus, your paper (route) may lead to a draft outline that would be divided into three parts: (1) Pros, (2) Cons, and (3) Recommendations. You may also want to think about the tone you would take: Do you want to conclude for one side or the other, or merely provide all the points in the message and not make a recommendation? If so, you may decide that you want to make an outline for the body of your paper that deals with (1) Historical Background on Uniforms, (2) The Case against the Uniform, (3) The Case for the Uniform. (Remember, you will also have a short Introductory Section and a short Concluding Section.)

As you think about your map over the next few days, you may realize that you need to do some research in the library or over the Internet to see what others have said about uniforms in professional journals. But you also may decide that you want to talk even more to others. You may decide that you want to ask all the patients on the ward on which you are doing your clinical sessions. Or you may want to ask all the graduates on the ward (if you can find time to do this during your clinical session). You may also want to ask further questions of your instructor and classmates, either in class or by e-mail.

Remember that the map does not need to be neat and tidy; it represents a brainstorming session, and its purpose is to get you to start thinking. Jot down one or two words to include *any* ideas that come to mind, even if you think they may not be relevant later; you do not have to use them all, but you might want to put in the word "shoes?" to remind yourself later to consider whether standard shoes are part of a uniform. You may want to put down the word "cost" to remind you to think about whether standard uniforms would be more or less expensive. You may want to put down the word "supplier" to remind you to think about whether the hospital or agency would supply uniforms (perhaps at a reduced rate).

EXERCISE 2.2   **Organization**

Look at the Brainstorming Map in Figure 2.2 (page 28). Drawing on the ideas shown in this map (which would have to be augmented by some library or Internet research), prepare the beginnings of an outline.

COMMENTS ON EXERCISE 2.2   **Organization**

Your initial rough outline might look something like this:

Working Title: "The Professional Nurse in the New Millennium"
I.   Introduction
     — general statement that the image of nursing has changed and continues to change and is influenced by visions of nurses by the public, the media, the profession, and individual nurses themselves

II. Body of Paper
     A. Past images of nursing
         1.   Old-fashioned images of nurses with starched uniforms, caps, capes, uniforms — the doctor's handmaid, the sex symbol, the martinet
         2.   Development of a profession
             •   graduate nurses, registered nurses, professional organizations (local, provincial, national, international)
             •   better education (degree nurses)
         3.   Were these images accurate?
     B. Present images of nursing
         1.   how does the public (and media) envision nurses today?
         2.   how do nurses themselves envision "the nurse" (are there stereotypical images?)
             — is the stethoscope one of today's "stereotypical symbols"?

        3. "career" versus "job"
        4. influence of unions
    C. Future images of nursing
        1. will there be a "general image" in the future? Does there need to be a separate and distinct image? Will there be more than one image?
        2. ???

III. Summary
    — statement relating the three sections back to the opening introduction and showing that the various images of nurses from the past and present will also affect the image of nurses in the future
    — try to end with a memorable statement, or even a quote

Note that this is only a beginning outline. As you do more reading and more research into the image of professional nurses (past, present, and future), the outline may change.

CHAPTER THREE

Common Errors in Writing

Common errors are simple, everyday mistakes that you often find in the writings of non-professional writers — and even in the writings of some professional writers. You may hear some of these mistakes daily on your radio or read them in the popular press or magazines. You may even hear them in conversation with your instructors or in lectures. Think for a minute, however, about the SMART elements: usage is affected by route. The errors that we describe in this chapter are elementary ones that you should not make in formal college- or university-level papers.

Frequently, these common errors represent things that you can *say* (use appropriately, even in formal oral communications) but that are not appropriate in formal written communications. You may have heard the maxim "Write the way you talk"; that piece of good advice tells you to avoid seeming too pretentious. However, unless you have learned to use correct grammar and to speak fluent and correct English, you probably need to make some effort to write slightly more formally in your papers than you normally speak. For example, many teenagers today routinely say, "Me and George are going to the store"; in a paper, this would identify the student as one who is uneducated and careless. You should also avoid contractions (e.g., *I'm, we've, can't, won't, shouldn't, it's*) in college or university papers — unless you are quoting from another source or reproducing dialogue. So, when you are editing your paper, you need to look for these everyday errors.

In Chapter 2, we described the steps of the writing PROCESS, concentrating on the need for you to **P**lan, **R**esearch, and **O**rganize your information and on how you begin to **C**reate a first draft. We also briefly mentioned the

41

steps of Editing, Shining up your prose, and Submitting your paper. In this chapter, we want to discuss in more detail those editing and polishing steps — the ones you do after you have developed and drafted the content of your paper to your satisfaction. In learning to edit and shine your assignments, you need to look, in particular, at common errors made in written communications.

Although this chapter deals with some errors in grammar, this text is not intended to be a basic grammar book. If you have been accepted into a nursing-education program, you are expected to have good language, grammar, and writing skills. You should have, as reference tools, a good dictionary and one or two good basic grammar texts on your shelves to help you as you edit, revise, and polish your paper. Just how basic or how advanced your reference tools should be will depend on your present skills as a writer; choose the kind of book you need now, but be prepared to look for more advanced texts as you gain better writing skills through practice, reading, and feedback from your instructors. Appendix B gives notes on and recommends some useful reference books that might appeal to you.

You need to correct the following common errors before you type up the final version. Allow yourself about an hour to go through the final draft, looking for:

- long, complex sentences;
- passive (instead of active) voice;
- weak pronouns and verbs at the start of sentences;
- long, complicated, or inappropriate words (jargon);
- lack of agreement of terms;
- lack of parallel structure;
- misused words;
- biassed language;
- unnecessary words; and
- inconsistencies in punctuation, spelling, and capitalization.

COMMON ERROR: LONG, COMPLEX SENTENCES

Communications today has become a science, and a great deal of research has been done into what Flesch (1960) has called "readability." Such research shows that people with high school and university educations are most comfortable reading sentences that average about 20 to 25 words. When a sentence contains 40 or more words, even people with doctoral degrees tend to get confused and disoriented, although if they are familiar with the subject matter, they can often follow the ideas. Clear words, logical flow, and good punctuation also help a reader to get through the maze. However, long sentences make readers tired and irritable. Do you want an irritable instructor marking your paper?

Reading your paper out loud often helps you to spot long sentences, although you can also find them simply by looking at the final draft. Usually, you can divide long sentences into two (or more) shorter sentences that convey your thoughts more clearly. You do not want to make all your sentences short; doing so will make your paper sound like a primary school assignment. Just take care that a sentence is not too long and that there are not many long sentences. Look critically at some of the articles you are required to read. When you need to reread passages because you seem to lose the meaning, you will usually find a long sentence as the culprit.

EXERCISE 3.1   Long Sentences

Try reading the following long sentence, which actually appeared in a draft report written for the American Hospital Association.

> In addition to their primary mission of providing health care and related education to the sick and injured, hospitals have a responsibility to work with others in the community to assess the health status of the community, identify target health areas and population groups for hospital-based and cooperative health promotion programs, develop programs to help upgrade the health in those target areas, and ensure that persons who are apparently healthy have access to information about how to stay well and prevent disease, provide appropriate health education programs that aid those persons who choose to alter their personal health behavior or develop a more healthful lifestyle, and establish the hospital within the community as an institution which is concerned about good health as well as one concerned with treating illness.

Try rewriting the message on a separate piece of paper or on your computer. Then refer to the following comments for suggestions.

COMMENTS ON EXERCISE 3.1   Long Sentences

That sentence has 130 words in it. You could rewrite its message in several ways. The 122 words in the following version are divided into five sentences (two of which use semicolons, which help to turn the sentences into seven distinct thoughts); thus, this version is much easier to understand.

> In addition to a primary mission of providing care and related education to the sick and injured, hospitals have four goals. First, hospitals need to work with local individuals to assess the community's health status. Second, hospitals must help identify target health areas and population groups for hospital-based and cooperative health-promotion programs; they then develop programs to help upgrade health in those target areas. Third, hospitals also must ensure that apparently healthy persons have access to information about how to stay well and prevent disease; hospitals must provide appropriate health-education programs that aid people to alter their health behaviors and develop healthful lifestyles. Fourth, hospitals must be community institutions just as concerned with good health as with treating illness.

The following passage uses a different format to break up the message and make it easier for the reader to follow. It contains 128 words in two sentences, but the message is broken into seven distinct passages and is therefore easier to read.

> In addition to the primary mission of providing health care and related education to the sick and injured, hospitals have six other goals:
>
> - to work with others in the community to assess the health status of the community;
> - to identify target health areas and population groups for hospital-based and cooperative health-promotion programs;
> - to develop programs to help upgrade health in those target areas;
> - to ensure that persons who are apparently healthy have access to information about how to stay well and prevent disease;
> - to provide appropriate health-education programs that aid those persons who choose to alter their personal health behavior or develop a more healthful lifestyle; and
> - to be an institution within the community that is as concerned with good health as with treating illness.

COMMON ERROR: PASSIVE RATHER THAN ACTIVE VOICE

Use of active voice in writing gives strength and vitality to a sentence; passive voice slows things down. Passive voice is when the doer of the action in the sentence is not the subject of the main verb. Communication research shows that passive voice is more confusing and tiring for readers. Consider the following examples:

- A splendid coach was pulled by six black horses.
- The bed was pushed across the room.
- My first visit to Well Known Hospital will always be remembered.

The first example is not a major problem for readers. The sentence is short and clear. Occasional use of such passive sentences is fine because they may give variety to your essay. The second example illustrates how passive voice creates problems that may be more serious. Ask yourself: "Pushed across the room by whom? Does the reader need to know this information?" In many instances, the reader does need to know such information; even if the reader does not need to know it, he or she might wonder who did the pushing and thereby become distracted from your real message. The last example illustrates the kind of problem that occurs when writers misuse the passive voice; the meaning of the sentence is not clear. Ask yourself "Remembered by whom?" The writer of that sentence probably meant "I will always remember my first visit to Well Known Hospital," although another meaning is certainly possible.

Some writers, including many researchers, tend to use (and misuse) passive voice in attempts to keep themselves in the background. In recent years, even researchers are advised to use first-person pronouns (*I* or *we*) when necessary and to avoid passive voice. If they do not, they may get into difficulty with the meanings of sentences. In some of your nursing courses, such as charting (a different route than an essay or formal paper), you may be advised to "Keep yourself out of the report." However, you can still avoid passive voice and keep yourself in the background. Look at the following two sentences:

- Some statistics were found to be extraneous to the report but were put into the appendix. (Passive — found by whom? put by whom?)
- Some statistics did not apply to this report but are in the appendix. (Active)

The solution is to use active voice whenever you can. Watch for passive voice when you are checking your final drafts and change it when necessary.

Note that passive voice and past tense are different. A sentence in the active voice can be in the past tense. If you do not understand the difference, then refer to this point in a good basic grammar book. Try the following exercise.

EXERCISE 3.2   **Passive versus Active Voice**

In this exercise, sentences are in the passive voice; rewrite each one in the active voice.

1. A memo to head nurses, advising them of the workshop, was sent by the vice-president of nursing.
2. A copy of each prescription must be sent back to the ward with the drug from pharmacy.
3. The agenda for the meeting should be prepared by the representative from clinical pathology.
4. The purchasing department door was left unlocked by someone; this made it possible for the computer records to be picked up by mistake when the delivery man made his rounds.
5. Fire regulations must be explained to each new employee during the orientation week.
6. As he entered the hospital, the chairman of the board was hit on the head by a flowerpot falling from the window ledge above the door.

COMMENTS ON EXERCISE 3.2   **Passive versus Active Voice**

Most of these sentences could be rewritten in a number of ways, but the following show some of the easiest ways to repair each one. Think about each rewritten version. Is the active voice better in all revisions?

1. The vice-president of nursing sent a memo to head nurses, advising them of the workshop.
    OR
    The head nurses received a memo, advising them of the workshop, from the vice-president of nursing.
    In the original sentence, the main verb is part of *to send*. Ask yourself "Who sent the memo?" In the first rewrite, the doer of the sending is in front of the verb. In the second rewrite, the verb is changed. The head nurses are now the doers of the verb *to receive*. Ask yourself "Who received the memo?"

2. Pharmacy staff must send a copy of each prescription back to the ward with the drug.

3. The representative from clinical pathology should prepare the agenda for the meeting.

4. Someone left the purchasing department door unlocked; this made it possible for the delivery man to pick up the computer records by mistake when he made his rounds.

   Note that we assisted you with this example because we put in the words *by someone*. But see what happens in the next example.

5. (Someone) must explain fire regulations to each new employee during orientation week.

   OR

   During orientation week, each new employee must attend a session with the hospital's fire marshal to learn the fire regulations.

   The original sentence was taken directly from Well Known Hospital's orientation manual. The problem at WKH, because passive voice is used in the original, was that no one was responsible for actually explaining the fire regulations! You cannot edit that sentence; you have to send it back to the writer and ask him or her to make it clear who is to do the explaining.

6. A flowerpot, falling from the window ledge above the door, hit the chairman of the board on the head as he entered the hospital.

   In this example, the flowerpot did the action, so this rewrite is in the active voice. However, the original sentence is probably better because it makes the content more relevant. So an additional warning is needed: do not become overly dependent on rules (even *our* rules!). Think SMART.

COMMON ERROR: WEAK PRONOUNS AND VERBS

Poor writers tend to rely too often on pronouns (rather than nouns) and on weak beginnings to sentences. Such writing habits take all the vitality out of a written communication. For example, a pronoun often fails to convey the correct meaning.

> Students watched as instructors demonstrated the correct method for injecting medications into an intravenous tube. This is a common technique that they will be required to practise in the laboratory.

The pronoun *this* is intended to refer to the complete sense of the preceding sentence, but on first reading the pronoun seems to refer to "tube."

Furthermore, the pronoun *they* later in the sentence can refer to either "students" or "instructors."

Sentences that begin with "This is ..." or "There are ..." — or with similar constructions (e.g., "These were ...," "There is ...," "That was ...") — are usually weak constructions and can be strengthened merely by editing. For example,

> There was a beautiful princess who lived at the edge of the forest.

This sentence would be better written as,

> A beautiful princess lived at the edge of the forest.

The solution is to use strong nouns and verbs. Watch for sentences beginning with the weak constructions and change them when possible. Many weak openings can simply be eliminated, as in the example above. Always watch for a pronoun (especially *they*, *it*, and *this*) at the beginning of a sentence, and be sure that the reference to the antecedent noun is clear. Try the following exercise.

EXERCISE 3.3   Weak Pronouns and Verbs

Edit the following sentences.

1. There are two things that really bother me: weak pronouns and weak constructions.
2. Once upon a time, there were three little pigs who lived with their mother at the edge of the forest.
3. There are a variety of walkers which provide support to those who are weak and have difficulty maintaining balance. Some of these have wheels, although others need to be lifted with each step.
4. The nurses at Well Known Hospital use a variety of brochures, checklists, and instruction sheets to help patients learn postoperative techniques. They find the brochures are helpful and often use them to make notes about questions they need to discuss with their doctors.

COMMENTS ON EXERCISE 3.3   Weak Pronouns and Verbs

Following are some ways to edit and improve these sentences.

1. Two things really bother me: weak pronouns and weak constructions.

2. Once upon a time, three little pigs lived with their mother at the edge of the forest.

3. A variety of walkers provide support to those who are weak and have difficulty maintaining balance. Some of the walkers have wheels, although others need to be lifted with each step.

4. The nurses at Well Known Hospital use a variety of brochures, checklists, and instruction sheets to help patients learn postoperative techniques. The patients find the brochures helpful and often use them to make notes about questions they need to discuss with their doctors.

Remember that this point is important in written communications. In oral presentations (a different route), good speakers often form a sentence with a weak beginning so that the emphasis comes at the end, when tone of voice can stress the point for listeners' ears. You probably remember that many fairy tales or children's stories prepared for reading aloud start with "Once upon a time, there was...."

COMMON ERROR: LONG, COMPLICATED, OR INAPPROPRIATE WORDS

Short, clear, simple, direct words are better than long, complex ones that may confuse, tire, or hinder the reader. In informational writing, simple words have more impact than complex ones. Everyday words are easier for the reader to understand — and usually they are easier for the writer to spell correctly! Complex words are often jargon (also sometimes called gobbledegook, bafflegab, officialese, or newspeak). "Jargon" is a derogatory term; it applies when you write "utilize" for "use," or "debark," "deplane," or "offload" instead of "leave" or "get off." Slang (e.g., "dude"), foreign terms (e.g., "a priori," "au courant"), and outdated words (e.g., "whilst," "amongst") can also be included in this category of inappropriate terms.

Note that jargon does not mean professional terms — unless, of course, they are not suited to your receivers. For example, "Are you suffering from an acute upper gastrointestinal tract inflammation?" is inappropriate when you want to ask a seven-year-old child "Do you have a tummy ache?" On the other hand, it would be entirely appropriate to write in the nurse's notes "The child shows symptoms of an acute upper GI inflammation." When you, a nurse, are writing for nursing colleagues or other health care professionals, you must use the appropriate words. However, it is wrong when you use words only to mystify or impress, or when you use terms to disorient or confound.

Often jargon reflects popular words used in the media and, especially, in advertising, but nursing has its jargon too. Examples include "hospitalize," "operationalize," "bedrest patients," "maximize," "paradigms," "therapeutic milieu," and "conceptual frameworks." We are not saying that you should never use these words, but think SMART. Sometimes you (the source) may want to baffle or buffalo your readers (the audience). Some politicians frequently do this! Perhaps in some situations, you want to use big words to impress, but you must also consider the impact they may have on the reader. If an instructor gets the impression that you are using terms only to sound impressive, he or she may start looking into your sentences carefully for errors. Another problem is that misuse of words — and it is easy to misuse complicated terms — always fails to impress. When possible, stick to strong, clear, accurate, basic English. Try the following exercise.

EXERCISE 3.4   Long, Inappropriate Words

Practise simplifying your language by giving shorter or easier equivalents for the words and phrases listed below.

utilize	achieve
attempt	ascertain
numerous	terminate
demonstrate	consult
purchase	reside
modification	explicit
subsequent	initial
accumulate	remainder
obliterate	indemnify
voluminous	endeavor
for the reason that	
her personal physician	
he totally lacked the ability to	

List three jargon terms or complex words that particularly bother you; then give their simpler equivalents.

1.

2.

3.

COMMENTS ON EXERCISE 3.4   **Long, Inappropriate Words**

Following are some common substitutions. Note the word *indemnify*. You should also check a dictionary for all the meanings before you substitute a word. Take great care when you use the Thesaurus tool on your computer. Be sure you appreciate all shades of meaning before you change words.

utilize	use
achieve	get, gain
attempt	try
ascertain	make sure
numerous	many
terminate	end, fire
demonstrate	show
consult	ask
purchase	buy
reside	live
modification	change
explicit	clear
subsequent	next
initial	first
accumulate	gather, get
remainder	rest
obliterate	erase, rub out
indemnify	repay
voluminous	big, large, full
endeavor	try
for the reason that	because
her personal physician	her doctor
he totally lacked the ability to	he could not

Three words that bother many instructors are "impact" used as a verb (use "affect"); "hopefully," which is almost always misused (leave it out); and "irregardless" (there is no such word).

Note that you cannot always substitute. In the list above, "voluminous" does not *mean* the same thing as "big," "full," or "large"; in use, it gives the reader a sense that the noun described has many folds and a great volume of material. In a way, it implies all three of the shorter words. However, you are using jargon if you use "voluminous" to impress your reader or listener when "full" would do. Sometimes you deliberately try to impress your audience with big words. Such use is still jargon — but it may be acceptable in that instance. But such use does not usually work with instructors.

COMMON ERROR: LACK OF AGREEMENT OF TERMS

Lack of agreement of terms within a sentence most commonly occurs when the writer uses a singular noun and a plural verb (or vice versa), or a singular noun and a plural pronoun (or vice versa), or a singular pronoun followed by a plural pronoun (or vice versa). Whole chapters have been written on this problem in grammar textbooks. The APA (2001) *Manual* devotes several pages to examples of this common error.

Look at the sentences below, which should give you some idea of this problem.

- **The data is collected by questionnaire.** ("Data" is a plural noun, so you need to write "The data are collected....")
- **The doctors always enters the hospital through the side door.** (Plural noun subject with a singular verb.)
- **The head nurse should take care to avoid sexist language in their quarterly reports.** ("Nurse" is a singular noun; thus, the pronoun "their" should be singular ["his or her"], or the noun should be changed to a plural form.)

These three examples represent the most common problems with lack of agreement in sentences. Usually, these are simple errors that you make while concentrating on creating the content in the first (or second) draft. You start the sentence one way, then change your mind about the wording halfway through. Unfortunately, if you do not correct the sentence later, it will be grammatically incorrect. In the editing stage, you need to read your paper carefully to pick up such errors so that they do not get copied into the final version. These errors may also represent poor typing rather than poor grammar — but your audience does not know that. If you make too many such errors in assignments, your instructors will get a poor impression of your abilities. You may think that such errors do not occur often — but instructors find them in about 25% of papers.

Watch for these problems when you edit. Reading your paper aloud during the final draft — as if you were reading it to someone — often helps you to spot these errors. Try the following exercise.

EXERCISE 3.5   Lack of Agreement of Terms

Correct the following sentences.

1. Everyone should bring a writing pad to their next class.
2. Marjorie and Lily, after spending the afternoon in classes, plans to spend the evening with their husbands.
3. The patient needs to sign a surgical consent form before the operation; if this criteria is not met, legal problems may arise.
4. For patients with HIV disorders, even a minor infection, such as sinusitis or flu, prove dangerous.
5. Spread of cancer cells by diffusion are prevalent in serous cavities such as the abdomen or pleura.
6. Careless disposal of needles and sharp instruments often result in injuries to hospital staff.

COMMENTS ON EXERCISE 3.5   Lack of Agreement of Terms

There are various ways to correct the sentences. Here are some:

1. Everyone (singular) should bring a writing pad to the next class.
   OR
   Everyone should bring a writing pad to his or her next class.

2. Marjorie and Lily, after spending the afternoon in classes, plan to spend the evening with their husbands.

3. The patient needs to sign a surgical consent form before the operation; if this criterion is not met, legal problems may arise. (The word *criteria*, like *data*, is plural.)

4. For patients with HIV disorders, even a minor infection, such as sinusitis or flu, proves dangerous.
   OR
   For patients with HIV disorders, even minor infections, such as sinusitis or flu, prove dangerous.

5. Spread of cancer cells by diffusion is prevalent in serous cavities such as the abdomen or pleura.

6. Careless disposal of needles and sharp instruments often <u>results</u> in injuries to hospital staff.

Common Error: Lack of Parallel Structure

One of the most common errors in sentence structure is a failure to keep all elements that perform the same purpose within the sentence *in the same form* (i.e., *parallel*). This error is so common that grammar teachers have a little symbol — // — that they put in the margin to indicate faulty parallelism in a student paper.

Parallel structure allows readers to follow a list of items within the sentence clearly and quickly. Faulty parallel structure confuses and annoys the reader. For example, the following sentence indicates a lack of parallel structure.

Mary likes swimming, golfing, and to play tennis.

The sentence lists three things that are objects of the verb *likes* — but the three things are not given in the same grammatical form. The first two ("swimming," "golfing") are gerunds, but the last one ("to play") is an infinitive verb. To be correct, they should have the same (parallel) form. When they do not, the reader does a double-take and has to reread the sentence.

Correct: Mary likes swimming, golfing, and playing tennis.
Correct: Mary likes to swim, golf, and play tennis.
Correct: Mary likes to swim, to golf, and to play tennis.

Sometimes errors in parallel structure occur in the words you use to introduce a series of sentences, as in "First, ..." "Secondly, ..." "Third, ..."; to be parallel, these words should be "first, second, third" or "firstly, secondly, thirdly." Be alert to this problem when you are doing lists (as in job descriptions). Reading aloud also often highlights this problem.

The following two common (but simple) examples illustrate lack of parallel structure and the ways in which the sentences can be corrected.

Wrong: The lottery winner liked his new computer, his new car, and new swimming pool.
Correct: The lottery winner liked his new computer, his new car, and his new swimming pool.
Correct: The lottery winner liked his new computer, new car, and new swimming pool.
Correct: The lottery winner liked his new computer, car, and swimming pool.

Note that repetition of words may be helpful to the reader, and the first two correct examples may be easier to read than the last one. Repetition, whether explicit or implicit, provides a similarity of structure so that the reader knows what is happening.

Wrong: Mary was both required to give the intravenous drugs and to make the patient comfortable.

Correct: Mary was required both to give the intravenous drugs and to make the patient comfortable.

Correct: Mary was required to both give the intravenous drugs and make the patient comfortable.

Parallel structure sometimes requires you to understand and use common correlative constructions, such as "both ... and" or "not only ... but also" or "neither ... nor." As you will recall from your grade school days, these constructions are bound to one another.

Wrong: Frank was required not only to give the intravenous drugs but to make the patient comfortable.

Correct: Frank was required not only to give the intravenous drugs but also to make the patient comfortable.

Sometimes a sentence can get complex and require two sets of parallel structure, as in the following example.

Wrong: I will examine context of instruction, subject matter, resources, teacher and learner characteristics and objectives, then end with a brief summary.

The two main parts of the sentence ("I will examine ... then end ...") need the conjunction *and*. However, the list is also complex, so the reader can only guess its meaning. The following are possible correct constructions.

Correct: I will examine context of instruction, subject matter, resources, and teacher and learner characteristics and objectives, and then end with a brief summary.

Correct: I will examine context of instruction, subject matter, resources, teacher characteristics, learner characteristics, teacher objectives, and learner objectives, and then end with a brief summary.

Note that the "extra" comma before "and" in a series (which we discussed in Chapter 1) makes the list clearer.

The following is another example of the lack of parallel structure.

Wrong: The objectives of the course are to learn to: identify common mistakes in language; learn to set up a manuscript properly; accurately edit papers; and familiarity with spelling styles.

The punctuation here does not help.

Correct: The objectives of the course are to learn to identify common mistakes in language, set up a manuscript properly, edit papers accurately, and become familiar with spelling styles.

Exercise 3.6 gives a few more examples of problems with parallel structure. If they do not help you to understand parallel structure, then refer to a good grammar textbook.

EXERCISE 3.6   Lack of Parallel Structure

1. The nurse arranged a physical examination, advised the patient about better nutrition, and then she told him how to change the dressing.
2. You either should go to the doctor's office or go to the hospital's emergency room.
3. Wet bed linen should be changed immediately because dry linen helps to prevent skin irritation and promoting psychological well-being.
4. Nursing interventions for metabolic acidosis include recording of fluid intake and output; administration of alkaline solutions as ordered; sodium bicarbonate kept on hand for emergency use; and safety precautions if the patient is restless, confused, or convulsing.
5. The procedure for preparing hot packs, either by boiling or steaming, is similar to that for hot compresses.

COMMENTS ON EXERCISE 3.6   Lack of Parallel Structure

1. The nurse <u>arranged</u> a physical examination, <u>advised</u> the patient about better nutrition, and <u>told</u> him how to change the dressing.

2. You <u>either should</u> go to the doctor's office <u>or should</u> go to the hospital's emergency room.
    OR
<u>Either go</u> to the doctor's office <u>or go</u> to the hospital's emergency room.

OR

You should go <u>either to</u> the doctor's office <u>or to</u> the hospital's emergency room.

3. Wet bed linen should be changed immediately because dry linen helps <u>to prevent</u> skin irritation and <u>to promote</u> psychological well-being.

   OR

   Wet bed linen should be changed immediately because dry linen helps <u>prevent</u> skin irritation and <u>promote</u> psychological well-being.

4. Nursing interventions for metabolic acidosis include <u>recording</u> fluid intake and output; <u>administering</u> alkaline solutions as ordered; <u>having</u> sodium bicarbonate on hand for emergency use; and <u>implementing</u> safety precautions if the patient is restless, confused, or convulsing.

5. The procedure for preparing hot packs, <u>either by</u> boiling <u>or by</u> steaming, is similar to that for hot compresses.

   OR

   The procedure for preparing hot packs, by <u>either</u> boiling <u>or</u> steaming, is similar to that for hot compresses.

COMMON ERROR: MISUSED WORDS

Good writers generally have good vocabularies. They know a large number of words and select the most accurate one to convey meaning clearly and succinctly. For example, a good writer would know (or look up in a dictionary) the difference between a dock, a pier, and a wharf. The primary meaning for "dock" is the area of water next to a wharf or pier; a "pier" is a structure that projects out into the water from the shore; a "wharf" is a platform built along the shore (i.e., parallel to the shore). You can take a walk along a wharf, but beware if someone advises you to "Take a long walk on a short pier" or to "Go walk on a dock."

As well, good writers have learned to distinguish between homonyms (words that sound the same but have different meanings), such as "rose" (past tense of the verb *rise*) and "rose" (the flower), or "hanger" (on which you hang clothes) and "hangar" (in which you put a plane). You are expected to have learned these differences before you were admitted to a nursing program. However, almost every writer has some problems; once you know what they are, you can resolve them or avoid them. Here are 10 words or phrases frequently misused in nursing students' papers — with some advice on fixing them during the editing and polishing stages.

IT'S VERSUS ITS

Many writers (we are shocked at the number) have a problem with *its* and *it's*. The following is correct: "Nursing has its problems, but usually it's wonderful to care for patients." The word *its* is a possessive pronoun; the word *it's* is a contraction of "it is" (or, occasionally, of "it has"). Many students complain that it seems odd (or illogical) that the possessive pronoun does not take an apostrophe, as in "nursing's problems," "boy's book," or "John's dog." However, in "his book" or "the dog is hers," there are no apostrophes. You need to think of the possessive pronoun *its* as being like "his" or "hers."

You can also use another rule. You should avoid contractions in formal writing (you can also avoid many of them in informal writing without any problem). Therefore, if you are polishing your paper, check each time you have *its* or *it's*. If you can substitute "it is" or "it has," make the substitution and avoid the contraction. If you cannot substitute "it is" (or "it has"), use *its* (with no apostrophe). In other words, the word *it's* (with the apostrophe) would never appear in your paper! Of course, if the contraction is within a quotation from another source, you need to leave it; just be certain that you have copied it correctly.

Please note that there is no such word as *its'*.

WHICH VERSUS THAT

An old pun says "Instructors are 'which-hunters' — because they so often cross out *which* and substitute *that*." The two words have different meanings, however; both are pronouns, but *that* is restrictive or defining, and *which* is non-restrictive or non-defining. In conversations (one route), *which* is frequently substituted for *that*, but the meaning is made clear from the way in which the speaker pauses (or fails to pause) within the sentence or from inflections in the voice. In written communications (another route), the words themselves, aided by punctuation, must convey the meaning. So, because the two words have different meanings, good writers need to know when to use *which* and when to use *that*. Consider these examples:

- The pharmacy, which is on the first floor, is closed on Sunday.
- The pharmacy which is on the first floor is closed on Sunday.
- The pharmacy that is on the first floor is closed on Sunday.

The first sentence says that there is only one pharmacy in the hospital and that it is closed on Sunday. In the second example, the meaning is not clear, but without the commas most editors would assume *which* should be *that* and make the substitution. The third sentence implies that there may be more than one pharmacy, but the restrictive clause adds defining information; it means that the one on the first floor is closed on Sunday.

The third example can be rewritten in a way that would make the sentence shorter but just as clear:

The first-floor pharmacy is closed on Sunday.

One good way to determine when you should use *which* is to read the sentence and see if it makes sense if you omit the non-restrictive *which* clause. If the sentence makes sense without the clause, then use *which*, but be sure to add commas around the clause to make it completely clear to your readers. If you cannot omit the clause, then change the *which* to *that*. In other words, be your own which-hunter.

WHILE

Many students use the word *while* incorrectly when they really should use *although* or *but* or *whereas*. The error is simple to correct. The noun *while* means "time" (as in "for a *while*"). When *while* is used as a subordinating conjunction (i.e., when it ties another clause into the sentence), it still has a connotation of "time" and usually means "at the same time as." The old saying "Nero fiddled while Rome burned" is accepted as correct; "Nero fiddled while I played the piano" is only correct if I know another Nero and we are doing a duet! A good writer therefore uses *while* only when it has a timely meaning. Note the differences in meaning in the following examples.

- While I gave the medications, the doctor wrote the orders.
- Although I gave the medications, the doctor wrote the orders.
- The doctor wrote the orders while I gave the medications.
- The doctor wrote the orders, but I gave the medications.
- The doctor wrote the orders, whereas I gave the medications.

It is worth your while to learn the distinctions between *while* and *although*, *whereas*, and *but*.

DUE TO (WHEN IT SHOULD BE BECAUSE OF)

The word *due* is an adjective, not a conjunction, and the sentence must contain a noun to which *due* applies. Misuse of the phrase *due to* bothers many readers, although its use in conversation and informal writing is becoming more acceptable. Can you appreciate the differences below?

Correct: The cheque is due to arrive in the mail.
Correct: Her late arrival was due to the snowy weather. (But this sentence is clumsy and could be rewritten!)
Wrong: Due to the snow, she was late.

If you do not understand why the first two are correct, you need to watch for this phrase when you are editing your final drafts. Look carefully at the sentence in which the phrase is used; if you can substitute *because of* for *due to*, then do so!

FEEL (WHEN YOU MEAN BELIEVE)

In most dictionaries, the primary definitions for the word *feel* relate to "touch" rather than to "sense" or "consider." Good writers thus tend to restrict the use of *feel* to the primary meanings.

Correct: Feel the texture of his skin.
Correct: She feels her way across the darkened room.
Wrong: I feel this woman is ready to go to the delivery room.
Correct: I believe (or think) this woman is ready to go to the delivery room.

MAJORITY

This word is also commonly misused in conversation and in many news stories; students tend to use it unthinkingly in formal assignments. *Majority* means the larger (of two) and thus means "more than half" or "50% plus one" or "the greater part." You cannot have "a 40% majority"; in this instance, the word should be "plurality" (or you could say "won with 40% of the votes"). The same distinctions apply to the word *most* in good writing; be sure that you mean "more than half" when you use it. Also weigh the use of *many* (as in "Many patients ..."). Try to be specific when you use these words.

BETWEEN VERSUS AMONG

In grade school, you were taught the difference between these two words. *Between* relates to *two* people or things; *among* relates to *more than two*. You and I might keep a secret between us — but, according to the old adage, if we each tell another person, it becomes more difficult to keep something secret among three or more!

AFFECT VERSUS EFFECT

Affect is the verb; *effect* is usually the noun.

Correct: Does a high pollen count *affect* you? What *effect* does it have?

Simply knowing that these terms commonly create problems allows you to check their use. If you have a problem with them, then avoid using them by substituting other words. For example, if you have a problem knowing whether to use *choose* or *chose*, substitute the word *select*.

TO, TOO, AND TWO

Many people never have a problem with these three homonyms, but studies show that their misuse is one of the three most common problems in business writing. (*It's* versus *its* is the most common.) If these words are problems for you, then consult a good dictionary until you finally achieve an understanding of them.

THERE VERSUS THEIR

The third most common error in business writing is the interchange of these two pronouns. The word *their* is a personal pronoun from the same family as *they*; *there* is similar to *this* or *that*. Consult a good grammar book if you have problems with this pair.

Exercise 3.7 illustrates a few more of these problems and gives you a chance to assess your vocabulary.

EXERCISE 3.7   Misused Words

Choose the right word in each of the following options.

1. The administrator said it was a matter of (principal, principle) with her to pay only the (principal, principle) on the loan and not the interest.
2. Joan and Mary (alternately, alternatively) checked Mrs. Green's intravenous line and monitored Mr. Smith's blood pressure and pulse.
3. Tim thought it more (discreet, discrete) to wait until he was asked for help rather than (flaunt, flout) his superior strength.
4. The drug had some (adverse, averse) side-effects, causing the patient to break out in a rash.
5. Rani (lead, led) the way down the corridor.

6. She gave the report to Grace and (I, me, myself).
7. She expects to be promoted (some time, sometime) soon.

COMMENTS ON EXERCISE 3.7   **Misused Words**

The sentences should read as follows.

1. The administrator said it was a matter of principle with her to pay only the principal on the loan and not the interest.
   (*Principle* means "a rule of conduct" or "a basic truth"; *principal* in this usage means "the amount borrowed, as opposed to the interest on it," but can also mean "most important, main," and "head of a school.")

2. Joan and Mary alternately checked Mrs. Green's intravenous line and monitored Mr. Smith's blood pressure and pulse.
   (*Alternately* means "by turns"; *alternatively* means "choice" — and it might be simpler and clearer to say "Joan and Mary took turns checking Mrs. Green's intravenous line and monitoring Mr. Smith's blood pressure and pulse.")

3. Tim thought it more discreet to wait until he was asked for help rather than flaunt his superior strength.
   (*Discreet* means "tactful or prudent" and implies using good judgment in conduct; *discrete* means "separate or distinct"; *flaunt* means "to display blatantly, to show off"; *flout* means "to show contempt or scorn.")

4. The drug had some adverse side-effects, causing the patient to break out in a rash. (*Adverse* means "harmful or unfavorable"; *averse* means "opposed or reluctant.")

5. Rani led the way down the corridor. (*Lead*, pronounced to rhyme with "bead," is the present tense of the verb to *lead* and is only pronounced to rhyme with "red" when it is used as a noun to indicate the chemical substance.)

6. She gave the report to Grace and me.

7. Either is correct, although *sometime* (an adverb meaning "at an indefinite point of time") is more common in Canada.

Common Error: Biassed Language

In recent years, good writers have had to be conscious of using biassed language. Such language represents stereotypes that unintentionally creep into writing and that may offend or even insult readers. Common biasses usually represent sexist language or deal with cultural, religious, or racial terms. As well, nurses and nursing students need to be aware of biasses in terms used to describe disabilities or health-related categories.

Nursing students in particular need to be aware that avoiding biassed language is more than just being politically correct; good use of language can promote social well-being and help you and others to have better self-esteem. If you refer to a patient with diabetes as "a diabetic" or to a child with epilepsy as "an epileptic," you can sound as if you are using a judgmental label. If you practise avoiding biassed terms in your writing, then you will also be more aware of them in oral communication.

Perhaps because 97% of nurses (and about 80% of nursing students) are female, female nursing students tend to make more mistakes with sexist language than other university students. Such habits are hard to break. Most female nurses tend to write "The nursing student must be aware of the needs of all her patients." The usually accepted alternatives for the sentence above are "The nursing student must be aware of the needs of all of his or her patients" and "Nursing students must be aware of the needs of all their patients."

Sexist language, like other forms of sexism, hurts. Nurses, because most of them are female, should understand the stigma of sexism and avoid using sexist language.

Furthermore, colleges and universities have taken strong stands against sexist language and have advised all faculty members to be alert to this problem. Your instructors will likely notice, comment, and maybe take off marks if you refer to nurses exclusively as females.

Whole books have been written on sexist language and how to avoid it, such as *The Handbook of Nonsexist Writing*, by Miller and Swift (2001). Style manuals usually contain a section devoted to sexist language. The *Publication Manual of the American Psychological Association* (APA, 2001), for example, has several pages on this (as part of a larger problem of "bias") and an excellent table that gives some suggestions on how to avoid it. If you do not own an APA *Manual*, locate one in the library and read this section.

A common way to avoid sexist phrasing is to make your nouns plural. Thus, you would write "Nurses are concerned about their work environments" rather than "The nurse is concerned about his or her work environment." Use of the plural also helps you to avoid the "everynurse syndrome" — writing as if there were just one supernurse involved.

The following exercise gives you some practice in noticing, editing, and avoiding biassed language. Being aware of this problem will help you to avoid it.

EXERCISE 3.8   Biassed Language

PART A

The sentences below use biassed terms. Try editing or rewriting them to avoid sexist terminology.

1. The head nurse should ensure that her nursing staff attend CPR drills once a year.
2. When an anesthetist makes his rounds the evening before surgery, he needs to check with the evening admitting clerk to see if she has the list for the day surgery.
3. Every student at the University of Victoria has his name entered in the main computer.
4. To be admitted to the unit, a handicapped child must be able to dress and feed himself.
5. Dr. Alice Baumgart, past president of CNA, has been named chairman of the HEAL Committee.
6. When the new wing opens, the manpower needs of the hospital will increase 10%.
7. The telephone repairman removed the manhole cover so that he had easier access to the lines.
8. The man and his wife were upset when they found the flat tire.

PART B

Following are some common words that are suitable if you are referring to one individual and the sex is known, but that are sexist when the individual is not known. Try to supply a term that would be an acceptable non-sexist alternative.

waiter, waitress
alderman
spokesman, spokeswoman
steward, stewardess
mailman
weatherman, weather girl

fireman
poet, poetess

COMMENTS ON EXERCISE 3.8   **Biassed Language**

There are several ways that you can fix the sexist writing. The following examples should help you to begin thinking about the appropriate use of words.

1. The head nurse should ensure that the nursing staff attend CPR drills once a year. (OR Head nurses should ensure that their nursing staff....)

2. When the anesthetist makes rounds the evening before surgery, he or she needs to check with the evening admitting clerk to see if the day surgery list is ready.

3. Every student at the University of Victoria has his or her name entered in the main computer. (OR Students at the University of Victoria have their names....)

4. To be admitted to the unit, a child with a handicap must be able to eat and get dressed without help. (This version avoids the tiresome "himself or herself.")

5. Dr. Alice Baumgart, past president of CNA, has been named chair of the HEAL Committee. (OR ... named to chair the HEAL Committee.)

6. When the new wing opens, the workforce needs of the hospital will increase 10%. (OR ... the personnel needs....)

7. The telephone repairer removed the utility-hole cover so that access to the lines was easier.

8. The husband and wife were upset when they found the flat tire. (OR The man and woman were upset....) Some readers find the phrase "man and his wife" offensive because it suggests that the woman is defined in a possessive relationship. The parallel structure of "man and woman" or "husband and wife" is preferred.

PART B

Following are some acceptable non-sexist alternatives.

waiter, waitress	server, waiter (waiter is often recommended for both)
alderman	councillor (councillor has been officially adopted by many city and municipal councils)
spokesman, spokeswoman	representative ("spokesperson" may be acceptable depending on your audience)
steward, stewardess	flight attendant (for unions, steward is used for both sexes; steward is also used for both sexes on ships)
mailman	mail carrier
weatherman, weather girl	weather forecaster
fireman	fire fighter ("stoker" is used for trains and ships)
poet, poetess	poet (poet is recommended for both sexes)

These are terms discussed fully in *The Handbook of Nonsexist Writing*, by Miller and Swift (2001). We recommend this book as solid reading when you have time. If you do not have time, then be aware that sexist terminology is not acceptable at the college level.

COMMON ERROR: UNNECESSARY WORDS

You should always edit out unnecessary words, leaving sentences tighter, crisper, clearer, and easier to read. In your first draft, you may write a sentence such as the following:

> An example of this problem is the fact that fever patients need increased rest and increased fluid intake.

During editing, you could rewrite the sentence as follows:

> For example, fever patients need increased rest and increased fluids.

Most grammar books contain long lists of wordy phrases. The following are just a few examples of phrases that could be pared down.

- in order to (just plain *to* usually does the job)
- at the present time (use *now* if anything)
- at this point in time (use *now*)

- the reason why (*the reason*)
- for the reason that (*because, since*)
- in the event that (*if*)
- are of the opinion that (*believe*)
- consensus of opinion (*consensus*)

Please watch for "in order to"; if you cannot substitute *to*, then the sentence may have a more serious problem!

Speakers (especially politicians responding to questions) tend to use long, unnecessary opening phrases to give themselves time to get their thoughts in order. Writers can organize their thoughts before they write, then edit so that readers can gain the essential message more easily. Watch for these phrases:

- It goes without saying that ... (then do not say it!)
- It is interesting to note that ... (is the rest of your paper not interesting?)

The word *the* is a special example. Many writers tend to overuse *the*. Obviously, sometimes you need to use *the* or your sentence will be unclear or ungrammatical. Do read over your sentences, however, and see if you can remove this little word. Look at the following examples:

- The staff at the Smithview Hospital set up additional beds in the hallways when the ambulances began arriving with the victims from the air crash.
- Staff at Smithview Hospital set up additional beds in hallways when ambulances began arriving with victims from the air crash.

In the second version, four of five *the*'s were removed. The sentence still makes the same point, but it is much easier to read. When shining up your final drafts, look carefully for such extra words and cross them out. After a couple of years of practice, you will not even put them in!

Clichés are worn-out phrases that have been used too often. Originally, these phrases created images that sparked a reader's imagination. When they become commonplace, they no longer do that, and you need to weigh their use carefully. Either come up with a more exciting descriptive phrase that will make your paper memorable or leave out the cliché entirely. Some of the more common clichés found in student papers include the following:

- the bottom line
- quick as lightning
- good as gold
- the whole can of worms

- pretty as a picture
- quiet as a church mouse

Clichés indicate that you are a lazy writer. Avoid worn-out phrases, and be original in your expressions.

You should also avoid lazy words that creep into your writing but that fail to make any impact on the reader. In our writing workshops, we have participants stand up, place the left hand over the heart, raise the right hand, and take the following pledge:

> I solemnly swear
> that I shall never use,
> in my writing,
> that terrible, four-letter word
>
> *very.*

Participants had a lot of trouble with that final word; they could not understand why we were making such a big deal over *very*. However, even years later, nurses tell us that they have become better writers because they took that pledge and that they still feel guilty whenever they are tempted to write *very*. This may seem simplistic, but if you, too, follow this rule, your writing will improve.

If you take the pledge to give up *very*, you will be forced to think about your vocabulary. And that means you will take a big step on the road to improvement in your writing.

Very is the worst of a long list of lazy words that weaken your writing. Others include *quite, rather, some, lots, many,* and *few*. Think about these words for a minute. How much smaller than small is very small or rather small? If you mean tiny, minute, microscopic, or infinitesimal, then use one of those words — or, in writing, just use small on its own. How big is very big? Gigantic, enormous, huge, 298 pounds, six foot seven inches, 32 billion? When you are speaking, you can use body language (e.g., raise your eyebrows) and tones of voice (e.g., drawl the word *very*) to convey meaning. In your writing, however, *very* just signals that the following word was not strong enough on its own. Substituting the word *extremely* is no better; you have just used a bigger word to get around the real problem.

Think, as well, about misuse of *very*. If you write, "She was a very honest nurse," does that imply there are degrees of honesty?

The correct solution is to use strong, accurate, descriptive nouns, adjectives, and verbs. When you go over your paper during the editing or polishing phase, look for lazy words. Try the following exercise.

EXERCISE 3.9   **Unnecessary Words**

Look over the following sentences and simply cross out lazy words that add nothing to the paragraph.

1. Nurses very often neglect to mention quite obvious hazards when they are teaching patients to walk with a cane.
2. The implementation of these findings has been slow.
3. In order to write well, remove all extraneous and superfluous words.
4. The day was extremely frigid. Rather than spend quite a long time dressing all the residents in their outdoor clothes to take them out for some exercise, the nursing staff decided to hold a dance in the recreation room.

COMMENTS ON EXERCISE 3.9   **Unnecessary Words**

This exercise was set up to help you find unnecessary words; almost all the sentences could be rewritten to make them stronger.

1. Nurses ~~very~~ often neglect to mention ~~quite~~ obvious hazards when they are teaching patients to walk with a cane.

2. ~~The~~ implementation of these findings has been slow.

3. ~~In order~~ to write well, remove ~~all extraneous and~~ superfluous words.

4. The day was ~~extremely~~ frigid. Rather than spend ~~quite~~ a long time dressing ~~all the~~ residents in ~~their~~ outdoor clothes to take them out for ~~some~~ exercise, ~~the~~ nursing staff decided to hold a dance in the recreation room.

COMMON ERROR: INCONSISTENCIES IN PUNCTUATION, SPELLING, AND CAPITALIZATION

During the editing and polishing phases, you should review punctuation, spelling, and capitalization. You should look especially for inconsistencies.

Problems related to inconsistencies in spelling style were discussed in Chapter 1, and this final review is a good time to recall them. While creating the message, you may read several books and journals. If so, you may carry the style used in your readings into your paraphrases, writing "a woman in labor" on one page and "the labour and delivery room" a few pages later. Note that *judgement* and *judgment* are both correct. Which is more common in Canada? In the United States? In Britain? Which is recommended in the dictionary you use? The APA (2001) *Manual* recommends that you follow the spelling used in *Merriam-Webster's* dictionaries, but many Canadian colleges and universities recommend that the *Gage* dictionaries be used as spelling guides. Usually, your instructors are not dogmatic about spelling style as long as you are consistent throughout the paper.

You also need to watch the style used in punctuation, another problem area mentioned in Chapter 1. You have to decide — based on Source * Message * Audience * Route * Tone — which punctuation style to use. For example, you need to decide whether to use a comma before the *and* in a series of three or more items — as in "We bought apples, oranges(,) and bananas." This is a matter of style, but in formal academic writing the comma usually goes in before *and*. In many journals and most newspapers, this comma is omitted. The APA (2001) *Manual* recommends the use of this comma; if you are going to use APA style, then watch for this point. You must be consistent in the way you use the comma.

In North America, the period (and most other punctuation marks) go inside the quotation marks — unless the meaning would be altered. As you create a rough draft, however, do not worry about the position of a period. As you do the critical review in the editing and polishing stages, you should look at the position of every punctuation mark.

Use of hyphens is partly a style matter and partly a spelling matter. Would you write "Nurses are concerned about a patient's *well-being*" (or use *wellbeing* or *well being*)? Think about the following alternatives.

- caregiver OR care-giver
- lifestyle OR life-style
- president elect OR president-elect
- postoperative or post-operative

Compound words take many styles: some are written as two words; some are joined as one word; some are hyphenated. Furthermore, some vary depending on their usage in the sentence (e.g., "The lab did an occult-blood test" but "The lab tested for occult blood"). The best tool to help you with hyphens is a good dictionary. You should decide which dictionary to use and look up the word. Remember, however, that when phrases are used in different ways, the spelling or hyphenation may change. The spell checker on your computer may not be helpful with hyphens; for example, most spell checkers would accept both "pre-operative" and "preoperative" as correct spellings, even within the same sentence.

- Public health nurses give follow-up care.
- Public health nurses follow up clients.
- Instructors often use role playing in their classes.
- Role-playing techniques offer students opportunities to learn in non-stressful (nonstressful) situations.

Most style manuals recommend using hyphenated phrases only when necessary for clarity. The usual problem is that students are not consistent and sometimes use a hyphen, then later do not use a hyphen in the same word used the same way in a sentence. Watch — and be consistent!

Another area in which students are frequently inconsistent concerns capital letters. You will face a number of decisions every time you write. For example, if you are writing a paper outlining recent changes in the organization of the Canadian Nurses Association, you might write something like the following:

> At the Annual Meeting of the Canadian Nurses Association in June, the Board of Directors voted to replace the Advisory Council formerly representing its 22 Interest Groups with a new National Nursing Forum. The board decided that the forum would allow interest groups to speak with a united voice on matters and allow better communication among the groups on issues such as Liability Insurance.

> At the annual meeting of the Canadian Nurses Association in June, the board of directors voted to replace the advisory council of its 22 interest groups with a new national nursing forum. The Board decided that the Forum would allow Interest Groups to speak with a united voice on matters and allow better communication among the groups on issues such as liability insurance.

In both the above passages, there are inconsistencies. Either style — one using an "up style" with capital letters and the other using a "down style" — is correct, depending on the decision of the writer. However, once that decision is made in the first sentence, the second sentence should be consistent with the determined style. Either of the following would then be correct:

> At the Annual Meeting of the Canadian Nurses Association in June, the Board of Directors voted to replace the Advisory Council formerly representing its 22 Interest Groups with a new National Nursing Forum. The Board decided that the Forum would allow Interest Groups to speak with a united voice on matters and allow better communication among the Groups on issues such as Liability Insurance.

> At the annual meeting of the Canadian Nurses Association in June, the board of directors voted to replace the advisory council of its 22 interest groups with a new national nursing forum. The board decided that the forum would allow interest groups to speak with a united voice on matters and allow better communication among the groups on issues such as liability insurance.

Usually, the decision is a matter of style. The most important point is that you need to be consistent in style throughout your paper. If you decide to use capital letters, then use them consistently. But should this decision about style be yours? As noted in Chapter 1, style can be affected by Source * Message * Audience * Route * Tone. In making decisions about style for formal student assignments, two important elements of the SMART way need to be considered: audience and route. Has your instructor told you either in class or in the course syllabus that you are required to use a certain style manual (e.g., the APA *Manual* or some other manual or style sheet recommended by your college or university as a guide for student papers)? If so, then you should use it.

Even if your instructor has not specified a style manual, the route itself may dictate that you use one. When you were in high school, your assignments required a certain form, but that form is not what is required at college or university. The level of papers rises, and you are probably not well enough versed on the style decisions required. Style for college-level papers involves many elements! Even if your nursing program does not require you to use one style manual, we still suggest that you purchase one and learn how to use it. If you can make your own choice, then we recommend the APA *Manual*. It will be useful in many ways. For example, one of the most important concerns with college and university nursing papers is how to treat references. In Chapter 4, we go over the most important of these concerns and give you the basics of style for the first levels of college assignments. However, a style manual is still a useful tool to own.

Exercise 3.10 gives you an opportunity to catch some inconsistencies in hyphenation. Try it.

EXERCISE 3.10   Inconsistencies in Punctuation, Spelling, and Capitalization

The following two paragraphs contain many common compound words or phrases. The paragraphs contain some repetition and some informal words, and they could certainly be edited to make the sentences stronger.

However, the exercise should get you thinking about style inconsistencies and especially rules for hyphens. Simply insert hyphens where necessary. You should also look for inconsistencies in use of capitals, and watch for a spelling mistake.

> The vicepresident (nursing) decided that it was time to upgrade her 10 year old, workworn computer system by adding an up to date hard drive with a builtin modem. She called a face to face meeting with the hospital's Computer Programmer and the secretary from the human relations department. She preferred meetings rather than writing one page memos or using email; as well, with a meeting she could obtain feedback.
>
> As her Staff arrived for the meeting, she thought how lucky she was to have such a hardworking group (not a donothing or clockwatcher among them). She said that her aboutface on computer replacement came when the old fashioned softwear system she had been using let two hyphens slip by her Xray vision. She said that she felt a loss of self esteem, and it was all downhill for the old fashioned system after that.

COMMENTS ON EXERCISE 3.10   Inconsistencies in Punctuation, Spelling, and Capitalization

For the corrected version below, we put in hyphens based on the use recommended in *Gage Canadian Dictionary* (de Wolf, Gregg, Harris, & Scargill, 1997). Other dictionaries or style manuals may recommend other usage. The only spelling error was "softwear." Although you could have elected to put all staff titles in capital letters, the use of lower case letters is preferred, is recommended in the APA (2001) *Manual*, and is easier to read.

> The vice-president (nursing) decided that it was time to upgrade her 10-year-old, workworn computer system by adding an up-to-date hard drive with a built-in modem. She called a face-to-face meeting with the hospital's computer programmer and the secretary from the human relations department. She preferred meetings rather than writing one-page memos or using e-mail; as well, with a meeting she could obtain feedback.
>
> As her staff arrived, she thought how lucky she was to have such a hardworking group (not a do-nothing or clockwatcher among them). She said that her about-face on computer replacement came when the old-fashioned software system she had been using let two hyphens slip by her X-ray vision. She said that she felt a loss of self-esteem, and it was all downhill for the old-fashioned system after that.

Summary

The final review of your draft is an important step. Usually, you need all your major writing tools (dictionary, style manual, grammar book) at hand for this review. And it can take some time, which means that you need to plan your assignments so that you allow time for this step.

Fortunately, you will get much faster with practice, and what are now definite, separate, time-consuming steps will soon become second nature. For example, you should soon stop writing "very" and start thinking about the most accurate word even as you write the first draft. You will be alert to parallel structure when you start to make a list. You will be visualizing your readers while you are drafting and therefore starting to make your language suitable to your audience.

You may think that all this sounds like nit-picking. Remember, however, what nits really are. If you do not pick them out, you end up with a lousy paper!

CHAPTER FOUR

References and Bibliographies

If you (source) are not an expert in a subject, you may need to substantiate information presented to the reader (audience), especially when your information (message) is controversial, theoretical, or new. Usually, you take information from a reliable source, such as a research report or an expert, and include it to support your views. To do this properly in a formal paper (route), you need to know how to find new information and to acknowledge, through references, the material you use.

References and bibliographies are essential components of college- and university-level papers. Furthermore, the need for good references and bibliographies increases throughout your nursing program. In your first-year papers, you may use only a few references, but you will use many more as you proceed through the program. Furthermore, on graduation, when you use evidence-based nursing in your work, you may need to use references on the job. If you decide to take a master's degree, you will need to be familiar with several styles of references and bibliographies.

This chapter is intended to introduce you to ways of gathering information for your paper, usually through libraries and the Internet, and to help you learn to use this material as references and bibliographies within your paper. It will also acquaint you further with some of the mysteries of style manuals. The summary here will suffice for most first-year papers, but you also need to consider buying a good style manual as a reference tool.

This chapter provides background information usually not included in style manuals. In particular, we:

- outline how to find information for your paper;
- explain briefly how and why a reference is used;
- comment briefly on plagiarism;
- introduce you to methods used for references (the numerical style and the author–year style);
- describe what a complete citation includes; and
- identify three of the most common errors in references that students make in papers.

FINDING INFORMATION FOR YOUR PAPER

Assignments at the college and university level almost always require research, so you need to be familiar with the resources available. You likely will have been assigned one or two texts for the course, and they should form the basis for your reading. As well, you should check out the topic in texts for your other nursing courses. Use the tables of contents and indexes to look for topics that you think would provide information about the subject in which you are interested. You may also find reference lists within these textbooks that refer you to other sources of information on your topic. In addition to your textbooks and lecture notes, there are many other places you can get information, including books and journals in libraries, Internet searches, and interviews and computer exchanges with individuals (these are called "personal communications").

LIBRARY RESEARCH

You should start by looking at books and professional nursing journals in your college or university library. If you are a distance education student, your program may offer special extension library services. Do not neglect other libraries, such as the public library; you might also want to check local hospitals and other health agencies, as some of these have excellent libraries for staff and allow nursing students to use them. The provincial nurses' associations and unions also have useful library resources. Some provincial nurses' association libraries offer "distance services" to student members; the library will lend you books or even send copies of relevant articles by regular mail or by fax. You need to check these out — and also find out if there are charges.

Spend some time in your college or university library finding out exactly what it offers and how to make good and effective use of its services. Libraries usually offer orientation courses at the beginning of each term; make the time to take the course even if you think you are competent.

College and university libraries usually have several types of computerized catalogues and databases, many of which you may use from home through the Internet. You must know how to use all of these to do literature searches. The basic catalogue provides information on books and journal titles available within the library; using this is usually relatively simple, with a choice of "menu" items such as author, title, or subject. Subject headings and keywords help you to find books even when you do not know the titles or authors' names. ("Keywords" are essentially the same kind of words or phrases that you use when you look for information in an index.)

You also should look for articles on your subject in recent issues of professional nursing journals. The information in journal articles is often more up to date than that in books. The reading list for your course may identify a few articles. However, spend some time looking for brand-new articles on the subject; keeping abreast of the latest research always impresses an instructor. Early in your nursing program, spend time in the periodicals section of your library finding out which nursing, medical, and allied health journals are available. Browse regularly in the latest issues.

Most libraries also have access to databases or computerized indexes for journal articles, often arranged by subject; these may be on separate terminals in one section of the library, but more often you can access them on the library's home page. For example, you may find that you can browse in "e-journals," which may contain the full text of articles; not all journals, however, provide full articles over the Internet, so dependence on e-journals may restrict your search. Instead, you should access specific databases or indexes. These may provide information based only on the abstracts, rather than the full text of articles, but they do introduce you to a wider range of relevant professional journals. One such database is CINAHL, which stands for "Computerized Index to Nursing and Allied Health Literature" and is the one most useful for nursing students; MED-LINE focusses on medical and allied journals; PsycINFO is an indexing service for psychology and allied disciplines. They will help you identify articles through the use of keywords. You also should check the subject guides on your library's home page; sometimes the librarians put together useful relevant information under headings such as "nursing."

As well as online services, public, college, and university libraries may subscribe to CD-ROM services that index and provide access to journal articles. One CD-ROM service is the *Health Reference Center*; it provides selected indexes, abstracts, and, frequently, full-text articles from approximately 2,500 journals, including 150 core health journals (e.g., *Cancer*, *Journal of the American Medical Association*, and *RN*, to name just a few).

If your library has these indexing services or CD-ROMs, you can use keywords to prepare an up-to-date list of articles on your topic from hundreds of journals. In some instances, you can even print out or copy onto a disk, usually at a cost per page, the abstract or the complete article. Even if you cannot print out the article itself, you can search for it in your libraries and read it there or photocopy it for use when you write your paper. Printing out or photocopying articles while you are at the library can be costly, but may save you hours of work later. But whether you make notes, make a disk copy, photocopy, or print out the material, be certain that you make full and accurate notes about who wrote the material, its proper title, and the place you found it. (There is more about this later in this chapter when we discuss how to do a "complete citation.")

INTERNET RESEARCH

If you have computer access to the Internet, you can reach libraries and, even more importantly, Web sites of health agencies and organizations all around the world. Most computer labs in colleges and universities, as well as many public libraries, have Internet connections. It may be to your advantage to do your searches through these computers rather than on your personal computer at home because the computer lab may offer technical assistance as well as being less expensive. Check into the facilities available to you as a student.

Be wary of the information you find on the Web, however, because you can encounter misinformation and poor quality research. Use your common sense about the authenticity and accuracy of the information before you incorporate it into your paper, and do what you can to check the validity of a site and its authors.

When you visit and collect information from a Web site, be sure you make complete notes about the author(s), organization, address, date you visited the site, and the titles or headings of the sections and pages you used to obtain the information. Because it is so easy to block and print or copy specific information from the Web, students often do not include the information that they will need later. Furthermore, many sites may be deleted or not accessible at a later date; check your Web addresses regularly. Figure 4.1 shows the information you need to collect for each of the online sites you use as a reference. You also need to note, if your computer does not do this automatically on your printout, the date you visited the site. If you were to record this information using APA (2001) style, you would state, for example: Received August 27, 2001 [use the date you searched the site] from http://www.cna-nurses.ca/_frames/resources/statesframe.htm

FIGURE 4.1   **Citation Information Needed for an Online Reference**

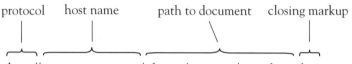

protocol   host name   path to document   closing markup

http://www.cna-nurses.ca/_frames/resources/statesframe.htm

http:// — the opening URL (universal resource locator), often referred to as a protocol

www. — the designation for a World Wide Web search

cna-nurses.ca/ — the home page address of the association or other author (in this case, for the Canadian Nurses Association [CNA]; the "ca" portion indicates that it is a Canadian address)

_frames/resources/statesframe. — the path taken to the document inside the home page

htm OR **html** — the abbreviation for "hypertext markup language," the closing item; be sure you copy it correctly

PERSONAL COMMUNICATIONS

Sometimes you will obtain information from a specific person; these are called "personal communications" and include interviews, letters, memos, telephone conversations, and e-mail messages. For a personal communication to mean something to your readers (audience), you (source) must provide enough information in your narrative to allow your reader to assess the value of this expert and the method you used to obtain the information. For example, suppose that you interviewed a clinical nurse specialist on one of your wards for some information for a paper. The following illustrate two ways that you could identify this expert in the body of the paper:

> A. J. Smith, clinical nurse specialist in the burn unit of Well Known Hospital, said an individual who experiences severe burns to a large portion of the body suffers profound physical and psychological shock (personal communication, December 5, 2001). She added that it usually is more important

during the emergency period to deal first with the effects of shock (such as loss of fluids and emotional distress) than to start management of the burns themselves.

OR

Individuals who suffer severe burns to a large portion of the body suffer profound physical and psychological shock, and usually it is more important to deal first with the effects of shock than to start management of the burns (A. J. Smith, clinical nurse specialist, burn unit, Well Known Hospital, personal communication, December 5, 2001).

Personal communications also include information received by e-mail. Instead of an interview, you may have sent someone an e-mail message asking about emergency care of burn patients and received the information in a reply. Some style manuals, and many instructors, suggest that you add the fact that this personal communication was received by e-mail to the information in the paper. You must also have made it clear in your message to the person that you wanted to use the reply in your paper; some people do not like to have e-mail responses or personal memos quoted in a student paper. Chapter 6 contains additional information about e-mail messages.

Once you have gathered the information, you need to know how to incorporate it and acknowledge it within the body of your paper.

CITING INFORMATION IN THE PAPER

In preparing an assignment, you may use a number of books, journal articles, reports, government studies, dissertations, and other materials such as videotapes, items from the popular media such as newspapers and magazines, and information obtained through the Internet or through personal communications. You must always acknowledge your indebtedness for the ideas and information you use from these sources. You do this by using a reference or by listing the information in a bibliography.

A *reference* is used in the body of the paper to show where you use specific information from a specific source; more information about that source is given in the *reference list*, which usually comes at the end of a paper. A *bibliography* also comes at the end of a paper, and a listing there indicates only that you read or used that article, chapter, or book as part of your overall preparation for the paper and therefore are indebted to that source in a general way. A reference also allows readers to consult the sources either to get more detailed information on a point of special interest or to verify your findings if the information seems incorrect or controversial. Thus, you need to indicate how the reader can go about retrieving the original material. You need to reveal not only who the expert is but also how to find the material.

Most of your references will likely be to recent books or professional journals, but some of them are hard to find without full details of when and where they were published. Some references (reports, theses, papers presented at conferences) are almost impossible to find without specific information. Because of these difficulties, there are various rules about the way a reference is listed so that a reader can find the information. Style guides or manuals outline these rules (along with other rules, mentioned in earlier chapters of this book, such as when and how to use capital letters, how to punctuate, and which dictionary is recommended as a spelling guide).

You use ideas or facts from your reference sources in two ways:

1. You acknowledge that the idea came from another source but paraphrase it (i.e., put the idea in your own words, which must be substantially different from the words used in the original version).
2. You give the idea word for word as a direct quotation.

Either way, you must acknowledge your indebtedness to a source. You need to make it clear that this was not your own, original idea but was thought of by someone else. You do this by indicating the source in your paper near the point where it is mentioned; this practice is referred to as "citing the reference." If you use information that was developed by someone else, and you fail to acknowledge your dependence on this information, it is called "plagiarism," and it is a serious offence in the academic community.

Plagiarism

Plagiarism — use of another person's ideas or words without acknowledgment — can have grave consequences. In some instances, you may be given a mark of zero for the paper or suspended from the course. You may even be expelled from a college or university for plagiarism. Usually, the calendar of your college or university contains a statement about plagiarism; you should refer to this statement. Many schools of nursing also provide new students with a handout stating the school's position on plagiarism. This is a matter of academic significance, so please take care in citing your references.

The most serious kind of plagiarism, sometimes called complete plagiarism, is submission of a paper written by someone else for you. Complete plagiarism also includes using the main ideas and large passages from one or more published works as the substance of your paper, even if you paraphrase the material and acknowledge your sources. Such practices generally represent attempts to cheat.

Using a paper that you wrote for one course for another course is also unacceptable, even if you have modified it and updated the references and content; such a practice is called self-plagiarism. In some instances, you can build a new essay on information developed in an earlier paper, but you should obtain approval from your instructor first and, if requested to do so, provide a copy of the original paper. The new paper must represent more in-depth work, take a new approach, and be significantly different.

A more common instance of plagiarism results from sloppy note-taking during your reading or research or from failing to understand how to acknowledge the material you used from these other sources. Take care when you copy passages from another's work, and distinguish both ideas and phrases used in the original when you make your own statements. Instructors may find it hard to know whether such plagiarism was intentional or accidental.

Because of the ease with which students can copy material from the Internet (e-mail messages, files from others, pages downloaded from the Web) and put it into their own files, they sometimes lose track of what they copied and what they summarized themselves in notes. Keep good records, and be sure you identify the original source on all the material you download.

Information regarded as common knowledge does not have to be supported. For example, if you have spent time in hospitals and have been fairly observant, you probably do not need to give a reference for the following idea:

The majority of registered nurses in Canada are women.

In your reading, however, you have found an article titled "Disproportion: Men in Nursing, An Untapped Resource," written by a nursing student named Matthew T. Davis and a professor named Dr. Wally J. Bartfay. It was published on pages 14 through 18 of the May 2001 issue of *Canadian Nurse*. This article clearly states that, in 1999, only 5.2% of registered nurses in Canada were men. And you know that your instructor would like you to be definite about such statistics. So you might decide to write the following:

About 95% of registered nurses working in Canada are women.

However, you have to indicate where you found this statistic. There are various methods that you can use to show that you derived it from the article by Davis and Bartfay, and where and how that article might be retrieved by your readers so that they can check your statistics or read more about it. If you are using the reference style most common in nursing you would use the following format:

> About 95% of registered nurses working in Canada are women (Davis & Bartfay, 2001).

Or you might write:

> Figures reported by Davis and Bartfay (2001) show that about 95% of registered nurses in Canada are women.

In both these examples, you are paraphrasing (rewording) material that was in the article. If you used some of the same wording from the article, however, you would need to put that information inside quotation marks, as in the following example:

> Davis and Bartfay (2001), using 1996 data from Statistics Canada, report "That year, 258,735 people were eligible to work as RNs in Canada; of that total 13,465 (5.2%) were men and 245,275 (94.8%) were women" (pp. 16–17).

Do you begin to see the differences?

If from this brief explanation you do not completely understand what plagiarism is and how to avoid it, then you need to do some more research into that subject. Ask your instructor where you can find the statement on plagiarism that is used in your college or university, and read it. A number of articles available on the Internet also explain and give excellent — and lengthy — examples of the various types of plagiarism.

An important point to consider is that *you* and your readers must be able to distinguish your own ideas from those you acquired in your reading and research. You also must organize your paper in an original manner, and definitely not model its content on someone else's work. And you yourself must be able to distinguish between your own words and those of others and know within yourself when you are "borrowing" — even if you paraphrase. If in doubt, acknowledge the source.

In the three examples above, we have shown you one way to acknowledge the information within the body of the paper. You will also need a reference list at the end of the paper (or, in some courses, a footnote at the bottom of the page) that will provide all the information your readers will need to find the original source of the material. But before we can discuss what to put in a reference or how to set up the reference list, we need to give you a bit more information about ways of citing sources in the body of the paper. In the next section, we discuss the use of reference styles and style guides, which were mentioned briefly in Chapters 1, 2, and 3.

REFERENCE STYLES

The most commonly used reference style in nursing is that recommended by the *Publication Manual of the American Psychological Association* — as we noted in Chapter 1 (where we were talking about route) and in Chapters 2 and 3 (where we were talking about preferred spellings, comma use, and other common grammatical recommendations). This *Manual* was written by the staff of the American Psychological Association (APA) mainly for the use of individuals who write articles for publication in psychology and social science journals. The editors of these publications wanted their writers to be consistent in the manuscripts that were submitted. The fifth edition of this reference tool was published in 2001 by the APA in Washington, DC.

As well as giving guidance on grammar, punctuation, organization, and spelling, style guides outline the rules you should follow in identifying the sources of information in your paper — the recommended reference style. These rules relate to the way you mention the reference sources both in the body of the paper and in the list at the end.

There are many, many ways of doing this — just as there are many styles of automobiles or shoes. The main purpose of an automobile is to provide transportation; the main purpose of shoes is to protect the feet; the main purpose of a reference is to enable a reader to find the original material. You need to know something about the various styles in use because you will see many different ones in your readings. For example, medical, chemistry, and biology journals tend to use reference styles that are markedly different from those in most nursing and psychological journals.

Generally speaking, two main styles are used for references:

1. the numerical style, in which a number — often a small, superscript number — is given within the text and the full information about each reference is listed at the end of the paper in numerical order.
2. the author–year style, in which the names of the authors and the year of the publication are worked into the text, either in parentheses or within the sentence itself; the reference list at the end then contains the full source information, with the items listed in alphabetical order according to the last name of the primary author.

The first (numerical) style is used in *Canadian Nurse*, the professional nursing journal published by the Canadian Nurses Association, and it may be the style that you were taught in high school. It is also used in many English courses. The author–year style, which is also called the Harvard method, is, with specific embellishments, the one recommended in the APA (2001) *Manual*; it is used in most nursing journals and is the one most often recommended in schools of nursing in Canada. Find out from your instructor which style you should use.

Drawing on the information about the Davis and Bartfay article mentioned above, an example of the numerical style is:

About 95% of registered nurses working in Canada are women.[1]

Then, in the reference list at the end of the paper, you would supply all the details a reader would need to find the specific article containing the information about the numbers of registered nurses; your citation would look something like this (depending on which style manual you used as a reference):

1. Davis, MT, and Bartfay, WJ. Disproportion: Men in Nursing, An Untapped Resource. *Canadian Nurse*, 2001, Vol. 97, No. 5, pp. 14–18.

If you were using the APA (2001) *Manual*, the information in the body of the paper probably would be given this way:

About 95% of registered nurses working in Canada are women (Davis & Bartfay, 2001).

The full information about the article in the reference list would be arranged alphabetically by author and presented as follows:

Davis, M. T., & Bartfay, W. J. (2001). Disproportion: Men in nursing, an untapped resource. *Canadian Nurse, 97*(5), 14–18.

Please look carefully at and compare the two examples of what might appear in the reference list. You will notice a large number of minor differences between them, such as the use of periods in the initials, the use of the ampersand (&), the way capital letters are used in the title, the position of the year the journal was published, the way the page numbers are given, the way the material is formatted or set up within the paper, and so on. All these are "rules" of style that depend on which style manual is preferred by your audience, whether that audience is your instructor or the editors of a journal to which you want to submit your paper.

Both the author–year and the numerical styles have strengths and weaknesses. The author–year method allows a knowledgeable reader to assess the importance of a reference without the tiresome chore of flipping to the end of the paper to see if the information comes from a well-known expert or from some esoteric source. As well, the reader can identify how recently the information was published or used; currency is particularly important in research papers. However, when many references are used, having the authors' names in the text can be tiresome for the reader. The numerical method is less distracting; the reader can concentrate on the message. The numerical method is particularly useful for short articles in which readers can quickly find the references.

How do you decide which style to use? Remember to think SMART. Have you been told by your instructor (audience) which style to use? Does the content (message) dictate the style? If you are writing for a newspaper or journal, what style does that publication (route) use? Which style do you (source) prefer? Notice which basic element we asked about first: audience. If your instructor has stated a preference, then you should use that style — or expect to lose marks! Check to see if this style is also used in the other departments in your college or university, especially for courses in the humanities or the sciences; other departments may recommend other styles. Many colleges issue a style sheet that all departments are required to follow.

No matter what style is used, however, you will need to provide the *full* information that will enable a reader (or even you) to find the article again. So, before you learn how to "do" your reference, you need to know what information constitutes a *complete citation*. Once you know that, you can apply the recommended style.

A COMPLETE CITATION

Earlier in this chapter, we suggested that, as you gather information during your reading in the library or your searches over the Internet, you need to put full information about the source on all the material you collect, whether it is notes or photocopies or printouts. In other words, you need to be able to give a full citation for all the material you use in your paper, usually either in a *reference list* or in a *bibliography* (we explain more about each of these later in this chapter). So as you read and review each book or article, make *complete* notes about its source.

Complete citation information includes

- the full names of all authors or editors,
- the date of publication,
- the complete title of the article in a journal OR the title of the chapter in a book *if* chapters are not all by the same author,

- the complete title of the journal or book (including the edition number),
- other publishing information, and
- page numbers.

Each of these items will be discussed separately in more detail.

NAME(S) OF AUTHOR(S)

The most important information in identifying the source of the material you have used is the name or names of the author or authors. Your readers (particularly your instructor) will want to know these.

You have to note carefully *all* the names given on the material you read and to note their order. All professions have a few well-known names, and you need to recognize the important ones in nursing. A few style guides require you to use the full first names, but most (including APA) call for only the initials of the first names. But it is a good idea to include the full first names of all authors in your notes or on your copies because you may need them some day. You will probably be annoyed when you find an important article written by eight or more people, but you do need to record all the authors. Some style guides allow you to shorten the listing of authors above a certain number, usually more than six. You do this by using the phrase "et al.," an abbreviation for the Latin *et alii*, which means "and others." However, we strongly recommend that you copy the full names of all authors.

The most appropriate place to find the names of the authors of the material you used in your research depends on the material itself. In a book, the best place to find the accurate names of the authors is usually the *title page*; avoid using the names as they appear on the cover because the names may appear there in a shortened form. The title page of the book is inside, often about three pages in, and contains the correct title of the book and information about the edition number, which you may also need. Other information on the title page includes the name of the publisher and the city or cities where this publisher has its main offices — but more about these items later. The names of the authors of a report or of a photocopied paper of limited circulation are often given only on the cover; there may or may not be a title page inside, so in those instances you do take the names from the cover.

Sometimes the entire book is not written by the individuals named on the title page, but contains sections or chapters written by others. Sometimes the individuals named on the title page are identified as editors or compilers, which means they determined the contents of the book and may have written some of the chapters, but have asked others to contribute chapters as well. In these cases, the names of the authors of the chapters usually will be given at the beginning of the chapter or at the beginning or end of the section. For example, in a basic nursing textbook called *Nursing Foundations: A Canadian Perspective*, written by Dr. Beverly Witter Du Gas, Lynne Esson, and Sharon E. Ronaldson (second edition, published in 1999 by Prentice Hall Canada in Scarborough, Ontario), there are a number of short vignettes about pioneer Canadian nurses written by Glennis Zilm. If you wanted to use material from one of these historical vignettes, you would have to acknowledge Zilm as the author of the material, but you would also have to acknowledge that this vignette (using its title) was in a book (using its title) written by the three main authors. This means you need to note and record the authors (and the titles) of chapters or sections as well as the main authors or editors of the book. You can see why it is important to make notes on the pages that you photocopy.

The names of the authors of a journal article are usually given at the beginning of the article; occasionally, especially in mass-circulation magazines such as *Time* or *Maclean's*, the name of the author is given at the end of the item.

Sometimes an article or book or report is produced or written by an organization or agency rather than an individual or group of individuals, and there is no name of a specific author or editor given. The World Health Organization in Geneva, the American Psychological Association in Washington, the Canadian Nurses Association in Ottawa, and the Saskatchewan Lung Association in Regina are examples of organizations that issue publications. For such references, use the name of the organization as the author. Be sure you get the name of the organization right.

For television programs, films, and videos, you often use the name of the director in place of the author. This means taking care to read the credits at the beginning or end of the material.

DATE OF PUBLICATION

After the name(s) of the author(s) of the material, the next most important item to note for a complete citation is the date the material was published. The date of a publication gives you and your readers an excellent tip on how valuable the information might be. For example, if you were writing an article that mentioned the types of medications that might be ordered for a patient, an article that was 10 or more years old would be outdated. On the other hand, as in the example of the Davis and Bartfay article mentioned above, the 1996 census information would be the latest available until

Statistics Canada publishes its information from the 2001 census (which might be in about 2003).

For books, all you need to include in a complete citation is the year of publication (often called the copyright date). This information is sometimes given on the title page and sometimes only on the copyright page (usually the back of the title page). Sometimes a book goes through several editions, and several years may be listed on the copyright page; generally speaking, you use only the most recent copyright date given in the copy in which you found the material you wished to use.

However, sometimes a book is republished and copyrighted years after it was originally written — and you may need to make this clear in your citation (and in your paper). For example, Florence Nightingale's *Notes on Nursing* was written and originally published in 1859. It has been republished many times since; one widely available facsimile edition was published in 1946 and is available in many nursing libraries. This might be the best possible reference for you to use in a paper on the history of nursing. But it could be confusing to some readers if you indicated 1946 for F. Nightingale (your readers might think there was another F. Nightingale), so you need to make the dates clear in your notes on the complete citation and, eventually, in the reference that you use in the paper.

For articles from periodicals (including journals, magazines, newspapers, regular statistical reports, and other documents published several times annually), you need more than just the year; you may need the month and day. For many journals, you can "abbreviate" this information about the exact date of a periodical; you do this by giving the volume number and the issue number. Because libraries often bind past issues of these journals, the volume number represents the number of issues that likely would be bound at one time. Usually, this represents a year, although some journals are so thick that they have two or more volume numbers a year. *Canadian Nurse*, for example, which now is published 10 times a year, is usually bound by year, and so the volume number represents the year and the issue number represents the month; thus, for the Davis and Bartfay article, which was published in May 2001, the volume number is 97 (this journal first started publishing in 1904) and the issue number is 5. Articles from professional journals often have the date, volume, and issue number on every page, so this would appear on any photocopies you might make. However, not all journals do this, and you may need to look elsewhere in the journal for this information. Usually, it is on the table of contents page, or on what is called the masthead, or, for some journals, only on the cover.

For information retrieved from other sources, you also need to be sure to include the date of "publication" or of copyright — and sometimes finding this is tricky. For example, you may have searched for information on the

Internet. Because the use of such reference information is still somewhat new, there are various ways of noting the date. Suppose you were looking for information about the symbols used by instructors when they are marking papers; you found that the University of Victoria had a Web site with this information and printed out a list of the symbols. If you want to use this information later in a paper, you should be sure that you record the copyright date (which is often at the top or the bottom of the home page or of the specific section) and a date when this material was last updated. As well as including these dates in your notes for the full citation, you must also include the date you retrieved the information; this latter is important, because frequently a Web site will be discontinued. Some programs automatically include the date and the Web address on the printout; if the computer you are using does not do this, be sure you note it on the copy.

Dates for films, videos, and such materials are given in the credits at either the beginning or the end of the program. These dates are often given in Roman numerals (e.g., MCMLXXXVII which is 1987); you may use either in your citation information, although the arabic style is recommended in the APA (2001) *Manual*. You may also use the date on which you viewed a live (not taped) television program, such as a news broadcast. Dates for compact disks usually are printed on the disk.

You also need to record dates for personal communications. This would be the date you interviewed your expert or the day the instructor mentioned the information in the class presentation. If the lecture material is not just general knowledge but must be attributed to the instructor as an expert source, you will need to include the date in your paper. So get used to noting dates!

TITLES

Even listing a title can be fraught with problems. If you are referencing a book, then give its full title. Frequently, a book is referred to by only a portion of its title (e.g., *Notes on Nursing*), but its full title may have two or more parts (*Notes on Nursing: What It Is, and What It Is Not*). The title should be copied from the title page of the book rather than from the cover because the two sometimes differ; the one on the title page is the correct one.

The edition number needs to be included as a part of the title. A first edition usually is not specified on the title page (and so you need not give it); later editions are. If a book is a collection of chapters written by different authors, do not forget to give the title of the chapter that you are using (as well as its author or authors). Sometimes the title page shows that this is a *revised edition*, which is different from a second or third or fourth edition; in this case you put the abbreviation in parentheses following the title but not in italics, this way: *Title of book* (Rev. ed.).

If the relevant material is from an article in a journal, then the title of the article is given as well as the title of the journal. Be sure you copy the full title of the journal correctly. Sometimes the name of a journal changes over the years. The original title of the official publication of the Canadian Nurses Association was *The Canadian Nurse*. In the 1960s, when the journal became a bilingual publication, its name was *The Canadian Nurse / L'infirmière canadienne*. In 1999, when the journal once again began to be published in separate English and French editions, the name of the English version was changed again, this time to *Canadian Nurse* (without *The*).

In most student papers, these minor distinctions would not matter; you could simply use *Canadian Nurse* and your readers — including your instructor — would certainly be able to locate the journal in a library. However, some routes (professional journals) and some audiences (including some instructors) want to see the distinctions, so you would be wise to note carefully the exact name when you are making notes about the material you wish to use.

OTHER INFORMATION FOR RETRIEVAL

In addition to those three most important items — names of authors, date of publication, and accurate titles — there are a few other bits of information needed for a complete citation so that a reader could find and retrieve the original information. These other items concern the place of publication or production, the name of the publisher or sponsor, and the page numbers.

For books, information for a complete citation includes the name of the company that published the material and the city where the publishing company has its headquarters. Usually, this information is contained on the title page of the book. You may find that the company's name is followed by a long list of cities; you do not need to list all these cities, only the one where the book was produced (usually the first one in the list), and you can find or verify that information on the copyright page. For example, some publishers have their major headquarters in the United States or Great Britain, but their Canadian books are published through the Canadian head office.

If the city is well known, you are not required to give the province or state, unless there is likely to be some confusion. For example, a few Canadian publishers are in London, Ontario; you need to distinguish this city from London, England. Almost all style guides now recommend that writers use the standard abbreviations recommended by the post office for province, state, or country. Thus, for London, Ontario, you would use London, ON; you do not need to put London, UK (for United Kingdom), because readers should assume that it is the major world city. You would put Oxford, UK, however, to distinguish it from Oxford, NY (for New York). You also need to think SMART with the cities. If you are writing in Canada for a Canadian audience, then you probably could put Saskatoon, rather than Saskatoon, SK; if you are writing for an American journal, however, you would be wise to designate the province.

How do you get the list of post office abbreviations? Many style guides, including APA, list the codes for the U.S. states. For Canadian provinces and territories, you can get a list from the post office and put it on your reference shelf. Your telephone book may also give these designations, usually on the same pages as the area codes.

You can use a shortened version of the publisher's name if the publisher is a major one. Thus, you could just put "Merriam" rather than "G. & C. Merriam Company." You will soon catch on to the commonly known nursing textbook publishers. Take a look at the references and bibliographies in a couple of your nursing textbooks both to see variations in style and to see what kind of information is most commonly used. If the publisher is a small house or a small agency, unknown to the general public, you may also need to give a full address, although this is rare in student papers.

You also need to identify the city and the name of the publisher for reports and other published documents. Often these are published by associations, such as the Canadian Nurses Association. Some of the documents you will use for your papers may be published by government agencies or departments, and styles for the citation of government documents can be tricky. For printed materials that are available only in limited forms, such as theses and reports by some small local agencies, there are special rules, such as including the name of the university faculty for a thesis or the full street address for a local agency. Again, copy as much information as you can about the sponsoring university or organization into your notes so that you will have it when you come to complete your paper. Include as much information as possible from the cover or from the title page and copyright page; when you come to use the material in your paper, you can then check on how to cite the information based on the style guide that you will use.

If you are taking information from the Internet, be sure you make full, complete notes on the Web address; sometimes this is included on the printout, but sometimes it is not. You also should make complete notes on — or print out — the home page of the source, which will give you information that may be necessary for your reference. For example, if you print out a section on "professional images" from a work that has the (fictional) address <www.amu.bc.ca/>, you might not be aware that the section was from a document called "Attributes of a Professional," and that the "author" was the Engineering Department of the Alma Mater University in Surrey, British Columbia; however, all that information should be in your complete citation.

For films, television programs, and videos, all you usually need is the city and the name of the production company (such as MGM of Hollywood, California, or Warner's in New York). Compact disks usually provide this information on the disk itself.

For personal communications, it usually is not necessary to give the name of the city. If you are using information obtained from a printed version of a speech, however, you would include this in the reference list and identify the organization for whom the speech was prepared and the city in which the speech was presented.

The last bit of relevant information that you should be sure you have for a complete citation is page numbers. This is especially important if you intend to quote from the material. Page numbers for books and articles are usually easy to find, even if you photocopy them for later use. Just be sure, however, that the page number actually appears on the photocopy. For example, the opening page of a new chapter in some books does not have a page number, and if you copied only that page so that you would have the exact wording for a quote, you would find when you came to complete your paper that you needed the page number. Photocopies from large pages, such as newspaper pages, often do not show the page number; if you photocopy from a newspaper, be sure to write the page number on the copy. A few books, such as small books of poetry or catalogues, do not have page numbers; in these cases, you must do a rough count of the pages (often referred to as "leaves" and abbreviated in the citation as l.), and pencil in the number on the copy.

So, you see, making the notes for a complete citation when you are doing your research involves a lot of details. Get into good habits early!

BIBLIOGRAPHIES VERSUS REFERENCE LISTS

Do you know the difference between a reference list and a bibliography? The *reference list* (frequently entitled "References" in the subheading) contains all the documents that you have referred to (cited) in the paper. The *bibliography* contains all the documents that you have read to help you understand the content even if you have not actually cited them in the paper. Both lists are based on the complete citation notes that you made during your reading and research for the paper.

Thus, you may need two lists at the end of your paper. A bibliography is usually much longer and more complete than a reference list and might include general texts or style guides. If you did not use ideas or information from any books or journals in the body of the paper (highly unlikely for student papers), you would not even need a reference list. You would, however, want to acknowledge the various books or articles that you reviewed, and so you would have a bibliography.

Graduate students preparing theses (route) definitely need to use both a reference list and a bibliography. Because journals (a different route) usually want to keep the lists in the articles as short as possible, editors generally want only a reference list. Just to complicate matters, the APA (2001) *Manual* notes that students may combine the two lists into one, which then is usually called a bibliography. If you combine the lists, we suggest that you use the heading "References and Bibliography." The two do not have to be combined, however; you (source) can decide to use both.

If you use the APA (2001) *Manual* as your style guide, you will note that the format style recommended for both the reference list and the bibliographic list is the same. Other style guides, especially those using the numerical style, call for different layouts for the two lists.

There is also another kind of bibliography — an *annotated bibliography*. This list can be set up using the basic bibliographic style that your instructor (audience) wants and that you would use for the reference list at the end of your paper. However, after each bibliographic entry, you provide a brief note (annotation) about the material that gives additional information for the reader; you may even include some material that did not seem relevant for the body of the paper. You also may add your own comments about the merits or defects of the material. Annotated bibliographies are frequently assigned in more senior courses and are often used as the basis for a *literature search*. A literature search is done by senior researchers and often contains not only an exhaustive bibliographic list of readings relevant to the topic but also a narrative report in which the writer compares and contrasts the information in the various readings and is able to come up with new conclusions. Even some of your early assignments in your nursing courses are an elementary type of literature search.

We strongly recommend that, as you do your reading and research, you begin to create a *working bibliography* of citations for your paper. Many writing texts and many instructors suggest you should do this on small file cards, and you may find this suggestion helpful. However, if you use a computer, we recommend that you list your sources of information using a style that you will use later in your papers — even if you modify that style for your own use, such as putting in the full first names of the authors rather than just the initials. By doing this, you will find that it is easy to integrate the relevant references into your paper later. As well, you can keep and combine your reference lists for several courses and refer to the file again and again throughout your nursing program. As added tips, we recommend that you start to keep at least a backup copy of your reference file on a separate diskette as well as on your hard drive, and that you update and back up your disk version frequently throughout your nursing program.

You can purchase software programs that will force you to make complete citations, help you organize your references, and actually create reference lists and bibliographies in a variety of styles. Although they are relatively expensive, programs such as *Endnote ... Bibliographies Made Easy*™ (from iSi ResearchSoft of Berkeley, California) can help you create and store up to 32,000 references in one database. Then, as you work on your paper and enter a code for each citation, the program will automatically create a reference list using one of the common reference styles detailed in the APA, MLA, University of Chicago, or other style manuals. Each time you revise your document, your reference will automatically be inserted. Such programs are useful for graduate students working on dissertations and for researchers carrying out major research projects that may be submitted to a wide variety of journals. We recommend, however, that you first learn the basics of reference style before you invest in such a program. You then should check with other senior classmates and ask about the best of the current programs. And you should be certain that you buy a program that deals with the latest editions of the style guides.

You can create your own database based on your reading. Box 4.1 shows references from a sample "working bib" that we have developed based on the examples from real literature mentioned in this chapter. Each citation is followed by short notes, some of which include quotations, to give you some idea of what you might include. The citations shown in this example are *not* in APA style, but contain additional information (such as the first names of the authors and the library call numbers). The notes shown here are just for a working bibliography for a student paper; notes for a complete literature search probably would be longer and more detailed. As your file grows, you can cut and paste your reference lists without having to check out the style manual each time.

At this point you probably should also take a quick look at Appendix A (page 175). This gives examples, using APA style, of most of the common citations that you would need for a reference list for a student paper. The examples in our appendix are based on real nursing materials and provide information on how to mention the reference in the body of the paper and how to list it at the end. Each example is designed to show some typical type of reference, such as (1) a book with one author or with more than one author, (2) a chapter from an edited book, (3) articles from professional and mass-circulation periodicals, (4) information from films or newscasts, (5) information from a permanent Web page, (6) the more common types of personal communications, and so on.

BOX 4.1   Working Bibliography

Annotated Working Bib: Nursing 101

(Note to Self: The citations are <u>based on</u> APA style, but contain additional information, such as full first names; check the style before pasting a reference into reference list.)

Canadian Nurses Association. Policy, Regulation & Research Division. (2000). Registered nurses 1999: Statistical highlights. Retrieved May 23, 2001 from http://www.cna-nurses.ca/pages/resources/stats/ salary.htm (Printout available in GZ files on "Images of Nursing")

    This one-page summary by CNA of statistical highlights uses information from CANSUM, the Statistics Canada Online Statistical Database Canada 2000, and reports and a press release from the Canadian Institute for Health Information (CIHI), 1999 (see also reference below). This is a great site for current information, and of course CNA is definitely a reliable expert source! Check frequently for updates. This verifies the stats in Davis and Bartfay (2001). It also summarizes other excellent stats, such as average age of RNs, education levels, provincial numbers, etc.

Canadian Institute for Health Information (CIHI). (1999). *Supply and distribution of registered nurses in Canada.* [NOT SEEN YET]

    Check for copy in Woodward Library. Mentioned on CNA Web site and sounds like a useful resource.

Davis, Matthew T., & Bartfay, Wally J. (2001). Disproportion: Men in nursing, an untapped resource. *Canadian Nurse, 97*(5), 14-18. (Photocopy in GZ files on "Images of Nursing")

BOX 4.1   **Working Bibliography (continued)**

Working Bibliography page 2

This article was written by a nursing student (third year,
Queen's U.), Matthew T. Davis, and his professor, Dr. Wally J.
Bartfay. This article uses data from the 1996 census and from the
Canadian Institute for Health Promotion (CIHP) to give statistics
on percentages of male-female RNs; the references are good. I
should check the original sources for more data on race and marital
status. The article clearly states that, in 1996, 94.8% of
registered nurses in Canada were women (in a table on p. 16).
Possible useful quote: "That year [1996], 258,735 people were
eligible to work as RNs in Canada; of that total 13,465 (5.2%)
were men and 245,275 (94.8%) were women" (pp.16-17).

Du Gas, Beverly Witter [Dr.], Esson, Lynne, & Ronaldson, Sharon E.
   (1999). *Nursing foundations: A Canadian perspective* (2nd ed.).
   Scarborough, ON: Prentice Hall Canada. (GZ copy)
   Basic nursing foundations text used in Nursing 103. Chap. 1
   contains a brief section on the changing image of nursing as
   well as background comments on changing demographics.

Nightingale, Florence. (1946/1859). *Notes on nursing: What it is and what
   it is not*. Philadelphia: Lippincott. (Facsimile edition; original
   published in 1859) (Available UBC Woodward Library WY.N6 1859a)

Zilm, Glennis. (1999). Jeanne Mance, 1606-1673. In B. W. Du Gas, L.
   Esson, & S. E. Ronaldson, *Nursing foundations: A Canadian perspective*
   (2nd ed., p. 4). Scarborough, ON: Prentice Hall Canada. (See above)
   There are 14 short vignettes on Canadian nursing pioneers scattered
   throughout the first quarter of the book, all by this author. Some
   of these would be helpful in the trends and issues course.

Updated: August 2001

Appendix A is not intended to be a substitute for the APA (2001) *Manual*; that 439-page book is an essential resource tool for students doing senior papers and for nurses who wish to publish. You may wish to buy one or to be able to have ready reference to it in your learning centre or library as you polish up the final version of your paper. However, our Guide does provide additional background information about references for those just starting to write college or university papers and for those not familiar with reading and writing research papers. And it probably will be all you need for most of your papers.

COMMON ERRORS IN REFERENCES

Nursing students often make three specific errors when they are doing the references in their papers: failure to cite the relevant chapter, inappropriate use of secondary sources, and failure to introduce quoted material into the paper in a way that does not break the flow of the narrative.

FAILURE TO CITE THE RELEVANT CHAPTER

A number of students make the mistake of referring to a book when they should be referring to a relevant chapter. If the whole book is by a single author or a group of authors, then one reference will do. However, today many nursing textbooks are compiled by one or more editors and contain chapters written by different authors.

The following is an example of an incorrect reference:

> E-mail references should be written with the same kind of care as a hard-copy letter or memorandum in all but the most informal of messages (Hibberd & Smith, 1999, p. 560).

Although your instructor can refer to this source and check your findings or get further information (the basic purposes of a citation), this is not the way that the author–year method is done.

In the example given, Judith M. Hibberd and Donna Lynn Smith are *editors* of a text that includes chapters written by them and some chapters by other expert authors. The information in this sentence actually comes from a chapter titled "Writing as a Managerial Tool" by Judith M. Hibberd alone and, as author, she is the only one who should be mentioned in this citation. Thus, the correct way is the following:

> E-mail references should be written with the same kind of care as a hard-copy letter or memorandum in all but the most informal of messages (Hibberd, 1999, p. 560).

In the reference list, the full citation, using APA style, would read:

> Hibberd, J. M. (1999). Writing as a managerial tool. In J. M. Hibberd & D. L. Smith (Eds.), *Nursing management in Canada* (2nd ed., pp. 555–574). Toronto: Saunders.

You may need to give a separate citation for the whole Hibberd and Smith book in the bibliography (or in a combined references and bibliography listing). The bibliographic mention of the book would indicate that you at least browsed through it and may have read several other chapters that were not specifically referenced. And you may have to list several chapters from the book in the reference list. Doing so may seem to make your reference list longer than necessary, but it represents the correct way to list material from an edited text. This method is clear for your readers, and it gives the credit to the real authors of the information.

CITING SECONDARY SOURCES

Use of secondary sources can create problems in student papers. A secondary source means that you are referring to a text (and its author) cited in another text, but you have not read the original version. *Occasionally*, this is permissible — but students should not do it routinely, and not without good reason. (The fact that you cannot get the original is often an acceptable reason, especially in student papers.)

A main reason you should not use secondary sources is that the primary source (i.e., the author you read) might not have used the original material correctly or might have used it out of context. When you also use it without seeing the original, the error often gets compounded. So either go to the original or cite the material correctly as a secondary source. Another alternative is to word the sentence so that you omit the secondary source altogether and use the primary source as the reference; you have to do this carefully and accurately, of course.

In the reference list, you give the full information only for the secondary source, but you make it clear in the text that you are citing from a secondary source. A good style guide tells you how to do this correctly. You may also need to note when the original work was published. The following illustration might help you to understand this point. In England in 1859,

Florence Nightingale wrote: "Bad sanitary, bad architectural, and bad administrative arrangements often make it impossible to nurse." This passage was published the same year in London in a little book called *Notes on Nursing*. This book was republished in the United States in 1860. You may have read a textbook edited by Judith M. Hibberd and Mavis E. Kyle in which a senior nursing administrator named Mary Pat Skene quoted this passage from Florence Nightingale. In your paper, you might want to use this quotation to illustrate that some common nursing problems have been around for many years — but you cannot get a copy of the rare Florence Nightingale book to check the original source. Thus, you might use Skene's chapter as your secondary source, showing it in your paper this way:

> Nurses have long recognized that poor conditions in the workplace can affect the kind of nursing that can be given. Florence Nightingale, in 1859, recognized these problems, writing that "bad sanitary, bad architectural, and bad administrative arrangements often make it impossible to nurse" (as cited in Skene, 1994, p. 159).

In the reference list at the end of your paper, if you are using APA style, you would then give the following:

> Skene, M. P. (1994). Workplace design. In J. M. Hibberd & M. E. Kyle (Eds.), <u>Nursing management in Canada</u> (pp. 159–173). Toronto: Saunders.

You do not have to copy the Nightingale reference from Skene's reference list and put it in your own because you make it clear in your text that you are referring to a secondary source.

"STICKING IN" QUOTATIONS

Be careful about "sticking in" a quotation, even if you believe that it illustrates your point well. Sometimes you can do it and the reader can immediately understand the logic behind the quotation. Most times, however, you improve the flow of your writing if you "lead in" to the quotation.

Here is a completely fictional example of a poor way to use a quotation:

> Nurses need to be able to communicate well. "All nurses need a master's degree in English grammar" (Zilm, 1923, p. 34). If nurses....

This quotation may mislead the reader. Are *you* advocating that nurses need to have degrees in English but using words from Zilm to back up your idea? The following helps to clear up that question and improves the flow:

> Nurses need to be able to communicate well. Writing fanatic Gwennyth Zilm (1923) even suggested that "All nurses need a master's degree in English grammar" (p. 34). If nurses....

You may have noticed in some books that each chapter starts with a quotation. This literary artifice dates back hundreds of years and is a good creative way to get readers thinking. However, that is a special literary device and usually does not have a place within a paragraph, in which each sentence must flow from one to the other in a way that the reader can follow easily. So when you use a quotation within a paragraph, make it clear how it ties in with the previous sentence.

The same reasoning applies when it comes to including the reference within your paragraph. If you always simply tack it on at the end of the sentence, it may not assist the flow. This is why the author–year method of citation allows writers to put the author's name into the sentence and follow it with the year, as in the examples above.

Summary

As you can see, preparing written assignments can be a tricky business! You need practice to understand how to find relevant materials and use references. You may also need some feedback about how you use references so that you can learn to do them better. One way of obtaining such feedback is to exchange a list of references with another student in one of your nursing courses and then spend a few minutes critiquing them for each other. You may be surprised at the number of important points you pick up.

As this chapter also shows, a style manual deals with many minor points. For example, a minor change related to the typing of a manuscript was decided between the third and fourth editions of the APA *Manual*. In the third edition, the APA *Manual* recommended that you should use two spaces after punctuation that ends a sentence; in the fourth and fifth editions, it recommended that you should use a single space after punctuation at the end of a sentence. The two spaces after a period was a long-standing tradition taught in typing schools. The use of one space after the period broke with this tradition because computers now set type in a new way. This minor point is something about which you can decide; most instructors will not mark it even if they are relatively strict about other points of APA style. If you type your own papers, however, you may wish to learn this new style.

Another minor, but fundamental, change relates to use of the *hanging indent* for entries in the reference lists. In the fourth edition of the APA *Manual*, published in 1994, the Association's editors changed from using the hanging indent to using paragraph style for items in the list, but they returned to the hanging indent in the fifth edition, published in 2001. Thus, you may see two styles of references, depending on which edition of the *Manual* was used as a style guide for that article or textbook. The hanging indent style, which is now recommended, looks like this:

Zilm, G., & Entwistle, C. (2002). *The SMART way: An introduction to writing for nurses* (2nd ed.). Toronto: Elsevier Science Canada.

The paragraph style of indent, which was recommended in the fourth edition of the APA (1994) *Manual* and used in the first edition of this book, looks like this:

   Zilm, G., & Entwistle, C. (2002). *The SMART way: An introduction to writing for nurses* (2nd ed.). Toronto: Elsevier Science Canada.

Do you see the differences?

Entries done in the hanging indent style are easier for readers to find and read than those in the paragraph style. We suspect that the change in the fourth edition related to the difficulties many users found with early software programs, where the hanging indent style was difficult to do and involved several keystrokes. Now, however, most software programs have simple standard strokes for the hanging indent. Be certain that you learn how to set up a hanging indent on your computer keyboard, as it will make typing your papers and keeping your reference lists much, much easier. Note that the APA (2001) *Manual* states that if you cannot do a hanging indent it is permissible to use the paragraph indent instead; however, we strongly recommend that you learn to use the hanging indent style.

Using references correctly is an important part of college- and university-level courses. In this chapter, we have tried to highlight the main reference problems that seem to plague student nurses. We have emphasized use of the *Publication Manual of the American Psychological Association* (APA, 2001). If your school of nursing recommends its use, we urge you to buy a copy and put it beside your dictionary on your reference shelf. Even if your school of nursing recommends another style manual, we suggest that you borrow a copy of the APA *Manual* and spend an evening browsing through this useful reference tool. The APA *Manual* has excellent background chapters on the content and organization of your paper, as well as on the expression of ideas (writing style and grammar). It also contains material on ethical standards in scientific publication, on ways to present statistics in journal manuscripts, on electronic manuscripts, and on bias in language. Spend a second evening browsing through the manual recommended by your school, and you will have an excellent background for writing all your papers now and in the future. Learn how to use the indexes in these manuals so that you can find information quickly when you are finishing the final draft of your paper.

As you do your reading for courses, take a few minutes and look at the writing style of the articles. Learn to read critically for style as well as content. A good style manual will be of use to you throughout your career. Good style is like good nursing — you do not particularly notice it when it is good, but you really notice it when it is bad!

EXERCISES

Exercise 4.1 gives you some practice with references and is followed by some feedback that should help you to recognize what to look for when you do references. You may be surprised at what you missed.

EXERCISE 4.1   References

Just to give you practice doing references and more feedback about specific points to watch, try using both the APA style and the numerical style in the following simple exercise. Imagine that you are writing a paper about students working together on a written assignment and you wish to include as a quotation the sentence "Collaborative research can be fruitful and rewarding." You found this sentence in an article in the February 1991 issue of *The Canadian Nurse*; you look on the table of contents page and find that this is volume 87, issue 2. The two-page article, which appeared on pages 20 and 21, was entitled "Whose Name Comes First?" and the authors were Lan T. Gien and Suzan Banoub-Baddour. The quotation was on page 21. The sentence that you decide to use as a conclusion to your paper is this:

> Although working together on written assignments can be time consuming and frustrating, one article on this subject concluded that "collaborative research can be fruitful and rewarding."

Show how this sentence would be referenced in the text and how the full citation should appear in the list of references at the end of the paper. First try using APA style as described in this chapter and illustrated in Appendix A. Then try using a numerical style.

APA Style
   Text Paragraph

   Reference Listing

Number Style
   Text Paragraph

   Reference Listing

COMMENTS ON EXERCISE 4.1   References

Your completed exercises should look something like these. You probably thought of a dozen questions as you began to work on this exercise, so you can see why you need to own a manual — and why managing references is a difficult task!

APA Style
   Text Paragraph

   > Although working together on written assignments can be time consuming and frustrating, one article on this subject concluded that "collaborative research can be fruitful and rewarding" (Gien & Banoub-Baddour, 1991, p. 21).

   Reference Listing

   > Gien, L. T., & Banoub-Baddour, S. (1991). Whose name comes first? <u>The Canadian Nurse, 87</u>(2), 20–21.

Some of the points to note here:

- Be sure the page number is given in the parentheses because this is a direct quotation.

- Watch the position of the period at the end of the text; there are many specific rules, but in this case the period comes after the reference.
- A capital is used only for the first word in the title of the article in the reference listing.
- Capitals are used for all the main words in the name of the journal (a proper name).

Number Style

Text Paragraph

> Although working together on written assignments can be time consuming and frustrating, one article on this subject concluded that "collaborative research can be fruitful and rewarding."[1]

Reference Listing

> 1. Gien, Lan T., and Banoub-Baddour, Suzan. "Whose Name Comes First?" The Canadian Nurse, 87, 2 (June 1991), p. 21.

This is only one example of a style using numbers; you may have used another that is acceptable. Some points to note here:

- The reference number used in the text could be in parentheses (1) or in brackets [1] rather than in superscript.
- The page number is not given in the text, only in the reference listing, and not all the page numbers of the article are included in this listing.
- The word *and* is spelled out in this style (*&* is used in APA style).
- The title of the article is inside quotation marks (some style manuals do not use quotation marks), and the first letters of all main words in the title are capitalized (again, this depends on the style manual).

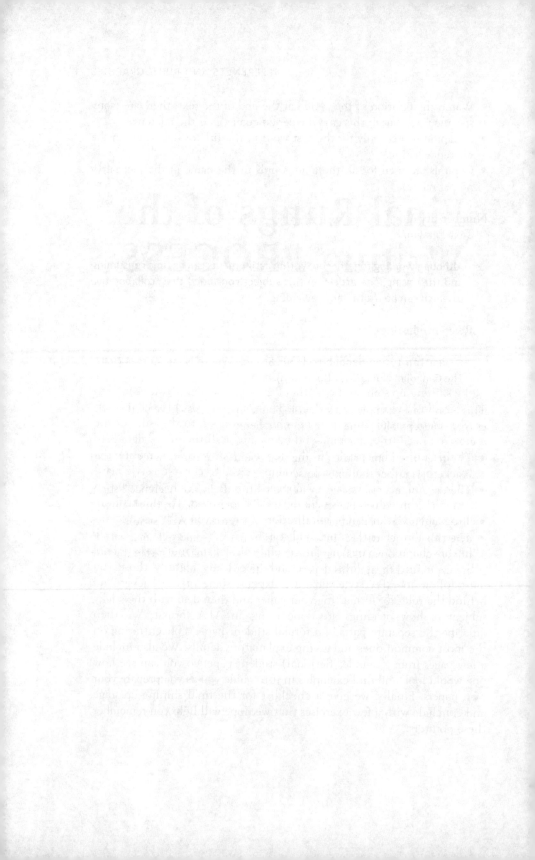

CHAPTER FIVE

Final Rungs of the Writing PROCESS

In the shining-up step on the writing PROCESS ladder — the second to last stage, just before typing up or printing out your paper for submission — you should ensure that it is presented according to the rules of the route. You need to understand and take care of all the minor details to make this a first-class paper. In this step, as when you were creating the reference list and/or bibliography, you may need to consult a style manual. Here you act as your own copy editor. As already described in Chapters 1 through 4, you will look for consistency in punctuation, spelling, abbreviation, and capitalization. As well, you will check details of presentation, layout, syntax, and style.

In this chapter, we outline the general rules of the route for a formal college- or university-level paper and specifically identify those you must follow in APA style. First we explain some of the background behind the rules for formatting your paper and then deal with the sticky subject of how headings are done using an APA format. We then describe the separate parts of a formal student paper, concentrating on the most common ones and giving explanatory details. We also include a few pages from a sample (fictional) student paper so you can see how one would look and find examples in it to guide you as you prepare your own papers. Finally, we give a checklist for the final shining-up stage and conclude with a few exercises that we hope will help you remember these pointers.

FORMATTING YOUR PAPER

Today's students may have two ways of presenting their papers to the instructor: by a traditional paper manuscript (hard copy) or, more recently, through an electronic file sent either through the Internet or handed in on a computer diskette. Most of the general rules for a student paper apply to the electronic route, so please read these first, and then we will comment on the minor differences if you plan to submit an electronic file.

PRESENTATION ON PAPER

Ideally, your final copy will be typed or printed on a good-quality printer; dot matrix printers often produce a typeface that is difficult to read, so be sure you produce a clear, readable text. If you are allowed to submit handwritten papers, take care that they are legible and follow these same general formats.

Most standard settings on the word-processing programs on today's computers conform with the basic rules of the APA (2001) *Manual*. You may find it easier to follow the APA guidelines if you do not ask your computer to "autoformat" but do the settings for headings and spacing yourself. Autoformat settings often use larger sizes of typeface for headings, something that is not required for a student paper. Take the time to learn how to set margins, to use the tab and indent keys, and to set headers and page numbers; such a learning investment will save you hours of reformatting as you work on your paper.

Note that the APA (2001) *Manual* has a short separate section (in Chapter 6) on student papers, theses, and dissertations. This section points out that you (source) *may* deviate from the guidelines in the rest of the book as these rules are for articles (a specific route). The *Manual* also stresses, however, that you should adhere to the recommendations specified by your department or instructor (audience).

Our "rules" and the sample student paper in this chapter provide a more complete set of guidelines for most student papers, especially those for your early nursing courses. Please note that rules for theses and dissertations differ again; guidelines to some of these differences are provide in our Chapter 6.

Select a standard typeface, such as Times Roman, Courier, or Pica; these typefaces or fonts have tiny lines, called "serifs," that help to carry a reader's eyes along the line. Typefaces without serifs (called "sans serif"), such as Helvetica or Gothic and most typefaces on a dot-matrix printer, are more difficult to read and cause readers (including your instructor) to feel tired. (See Box 5.1.) Use a standard font size; the APA (2001) *Manual* recommends 12 point. Use the same size throughout the paper, including in headings and subheadings; do not change font sizes for those, except *perhaps* on the title page. The APA recommendations for *articles* call for the title page to be typed using the standard font, but note that requirements for preliminary pages, including the title page, vary among institutions. So you could, provided your instructor allows this, use a larger type for the title on the title page. Some beginning students reduce or enlarge the font size or the line spacing in the body of the paper to help them meet the length requirements asked for by the instructor in the assignment guidelines; take care, because instructors are familiar with this trick.

Use margins of at least one inch at the top, bottom, and left and right sides of the page. These standard margins are usually programmed into your word processor or computer, although you can change them. One-inch margins allow your instructor room to write notes and comments on the paper. Occasionally, your instructor will ask you to leave wider margins so that he or she can provide more feedback. As always, an instructor's special requirements override all other style guidelines.

Double-space lines (even for handwritten papers) in the body of the paper; doing so makes it easy to read. Because your paper is a finished product in itself, and not a manuscript being submitted to a publisher for typesetting, you may choose to use single spacing for some parts of your paper. The APA (2001) *Manual* advises that you may use single spacing in tables, footnotes, and long quotations. You may also use single spacing in your references and/or bibliography (although you must then double-space between entries to make it easy for the reader to see each one separately). Generally speaking, double spacing in the reference lists is easier to read, so you may want to use it there as well. You may also choose to leave a space (double-double-space) before subheadings and in other places where it would improve the appearance of your paper (e.g., on the title page, after a title or a table, and before footnotes, or to avoid having a subheading on the bottom line of a page).

Number your pages in the top right-hand corner, using arabic numbers, beginning with the title page. In the section on student papers, the APA (2001) *Manual* notes that the preliminary pages *may* be numbered with lower-case Roman numerals (as is done in the front of this book); arabic

BOX 5.1   Serif and Sans Serif Fonts

```
Courier is a typeface with serifs.
Letter Gothic is a sans serif typeface.
```

numbering starts with a 1 on the first page of the body of the paper. This usually is not done with short student assignment papers, but is done with theses and dissertations. In the sample student paper that follows, we have numbered the pages with arabic numbers starting with the title page. We also suppressed the page number on the title page, because, in line with the APA guidelines, we thought it would look more professional.

You should also use a "header" or "running head," which is identified on your title page, in the top right-hand corner of each page five spaces to the left of or immediately above the page number. These headers are useful in case pages of an assignment become separated during marking or mixed with another student's paper. A header usually consists of the first two or three words of the title of your paper. You should avoid using your name as the header (unless your instructor requests otherwise); some instructors prefer to mark papers without knowing the student's name, and later in your career, when you submit articles to journals, they are reviewed anonymously.

Indent the first line of every paragraph five to seven spaces or one-half inch; on a typewriter or computer, this is best done using the tab key. Certain passages in the text, such as long quotations (i.e., block quotations) and some lists, may also need to be indented; this is best done using the indent key or keys.

Note that the APA (2001) *Manual* does not provide guidelines for indenting the annotations in an annotated bibliography (see Chapter 4), but its own annotated reference list uses a standard five-space indent followed by another two-space indent; in other words, the annotation is indented farther than the second line of the reference. This usually involves changing the spacing of the tab keys on your word-processing program. You *may* do this, or you may simply use two five-space indents, which is the common default setting for tabs on your program. (See Appendix B for yet another way to format annotated bibliographies.)

ELECTRONIC PRESENTATION

Many instructors now allow students to submit papers electronically by file transfer over the Internet or to hand in a diskette copy. Some instructors prefer to mark papers on the computer, as this allows them to give you a special kind of feedback, perhaps using a yellow highlight to identify specific passages that you need to work on or to redline (cross out) unnecessary words or phases. However, most instructors still prefer hard copy, and almost all instructors (except in some graduate programs or distance education programs) accept paper (hard copy) presentations.

If you and your instructor agree to the submission of an electronic file, check well before the paper is due to be certain you can send a file and receive it back. Many home computers, especially those that are a few years old, will not send and receive files in a compatible format. If either you or your instructor cannot read the file, you may be able to send it from the learning centre or library, as those computers are regularly updated and upgraded.

You may also find that there are some problems if you use e-mail to transmit a paper (through the cut-and-paste method); e-mail transmissions often alter the format, especially in relation to lines. Check the course syllabus and instructions and discuss electronic submissions fully with an instructor before assuming you can submit an electronic file at the last minute before the deadline. And always remember to keep a backup copy of your finished file.

HEADINGS

Headings are another matter of style that may differ in student papers. The APA (2001) *Manual* describes five levels of headings that may be necessary in articles. These are guidelines, and an author may select the level of heading that most suits the content of the article. The first four levels recommended by APA for manuscripts submitted to APA journals are shown in Box 5.2.

Notice that the APA style for articles (route) does not use boldface for the headings; the decisions to use boldface type or to change the size and location of the headings is left to the editors of the journal when the manuscript has been accepted. Notice, too, that, as we mentioned earlier, you may substitute underlining for italics in your headings.

The APA *Manual* says that three or four levels of headings should be enough for most articles. In some special research papers or in a thesis, a fifth level may be necessary; in these cases, you should refer to the manual. Notice that some text follows each heading; only rarely are headings set together without some intervening text. Usually, two subheadings follow one another only within tables.

Most student papers are relatively short and need only two or three levels of headings. You may also decide to use extra line spaces before headings and to put the headings into **bold** or <u>underlined</u> type to make them stand out. See the pages showing the sample student paper, Box 5.3.

PARTS OF A PAPER (INCLUDING A SAMPLE STUDENT PAPER)

A formal student essay may contain some or all of these elements:

- cover page (or title page);
- table of contents or outline page;
- abstract;

- main text or body of paper (but remember that the text of a student paper almost always contains an introduction, body [with its two, three, or four main parts], and conclusion, as explained in Chapter 2);
- references;
- bibliography;
- appendix or appendices.

BOX 5.2   Headings

Level One Headings

This is the primary heading that would be used, for example, for the title of the article. It is usually used only once in an article. Notice that it is centred and that the initial letters of the main words are capitalized. In student papers, this heading could be set in boldface. Bold letters are not used in manuscripts submitted to journals using APA format because editors determine the font that should be used for the title; think about articles that you have seen in journals and you will recall that many of these titles are set in large type.

Level Two Headings

Level two headings are centred and italicized or underlined. Notice that the initial letters of all main words are capitalized. Note also that there is no extra line of space (i.e., a quadruple space) between the sections in the article.

Level Three Headings

The third level is set at the left-hand margin of the page above the indented paragraph and is italicized or underlined. Again, initial letters are capitalized, and no extra line of space is used.

Level four headings. This level is also known as a paragraph heading. It is indented (using the tab key) the same distance as a paragraph, and the remaining part of the paragraph continues. Notice the sentence-type capitalization.

Many student papers, especially first-year papers, need only a cover page, the main text, and a reference list (or combined references and bibliography). On the other hand, a master's thesis requires a title page, approval page, acknowledgments, table of contents, lists of tables and/or figures, abstract, body of the thesis (usually divided into several chapters), appendices, and separate references and bibliography; it may also include a foreword and a preface, which come before the main body of the thesis, and an index, which comes at the end.

How do you determine what is needed? First, check the course syllabus for instructions about the assignment; most instructors state their requirements there. If you are in doubt, ask during one of the classes. Remember to think SMART.

COVER PAGE

One of the most important items in the final draft of your paper is a good cover page or cover sheet. Sometimes called a title page, it goes at the front of your assignment. It is often a good idea to begin work on your title page — or at least on the title itself — as soon as you begin to plan your paper.

On the final draft of the cover page (during the shining-up stage), you should include some basic information: the title of your paper, your name, your student number, the name of the course (and section, if the course is divided into sections), the name of the university, and your instructor's name. If you are taking the course through a distance education program, your address is also essential. Inclusion of your address is a sound idea for on-campus students as well, because occasionally an instructor needs to mail back an assignment (e.g., the final assignment of the year). You may wish to include your phone number or e-mail address; some instructors may comment on your paper or provide additional feedback if you make it easy for them.

A catchy title is a great idea. It introduces your assignment and can provide, in a brief phrase or two, a capsule comment on your topic. The title should be clear and interesting. You may also want to include a subtitle. For example:

Right Ways to Write:
Better Papers Mean Better Grades

Some instructors provide you with information in the course syllabus on what they want or expect on the cover sheet. If your instructor does so, then follow that style.

You may wish to develop your own style for the cover page. Just be sure to include all the essentials. And, even if you are a wonder on the computer and can develop a colorful cover with different, large, beautiful fonts and borders, remember that this is a student paper, not a document for sale. Fancy typefaces and graphics may give a different tone than you intended; some instructors do not like to receive a paper that looks as if you spent more time designing the cover than working on the content!

A sample cover sheet — a plain, simple one — is shown in Box 5.3 on page 116. You may decide to format your cover differently, perhaps using single spacing for the address, but this style is offered as a model.

TABLE OF CONTENTS PAGE/OUTLINE

In short student papers, usually a table of contents page is not required. However, many nursing instructors ask students to submit a table of contents or an outline — and that is because instructors know the importance of the O in the writing PROCESS; they want students to get into the habit of organizing and outlining. Furthermore, if your ideas do not flow smoothly from one section to another of the paper, a table of contents or outline helps the instructor to see your overall plan. In Box 5.3, the Sample Student Paper, both a table of contents page and an outline page are shown.

ABSTRACT

An abstract is a short, comprehensive summary of your paper. For journal articles, the APA (2001) *Manual* recommends a maximum of 120 words. Some journals restrict the length to 75 to 100 words. An abstract is an essential component of most journal articles, and you will see many of them in your readings; it tells readers what your article is about, what your conclusions are (briefly), and how these findings may be interpreted. Its main purpose is to assist researchers when they do literature searches and must review hundreds of articles. Abstracts often are included in online databases; potential readers can then usually tell whether they wish to obtain the whole article and read it.

Some instructors, particularly those in senior years, ask students to write abstracts as a learning experience. The APA (2001) *Manual* devotes a section to describing what an abstract is; refer to that as a starting point if you are asked to write an abstract. See also Appendix B: "Annotated References and Bibliography: Useful Readings/Reference Tools," which identifies books that have information on how to write abstracts. And you should search the Internet for articles and advice on abstracts — but remember to think SMART, and consider your *audience* and *route*.

BOX 5.3   Sample Student Paper

The following pages show portions of a fictional student paper to illustrate one way that you might set up a short and relatively simple paper for your instructor. Remember, however, that you must think SMART. Some instructors (audience) might ask for different layouts. The information presented in some papers (message) might call for a more complex format (e.g., more subheads) for the pages. If you are thoroughly familiar with APA style, you (source) might wish to amend this layout slightly to fit with your views about a good presentation.

The following paper was written in response to this fictional request:

Assignment 2 (due December 8, 2002)

Write a brief essay (about 1,500 words or maximum 7 pages of text) in which you recommend reference books that would be helpful to first-year nursing students. Use the *Publication Manual of the American Psychological Association* (5th ed.) (APA, 2001) as a guide for formatting your paper. Please supply an outline and table of contents.

BOX 5.3   Sample Student Paper (continued)

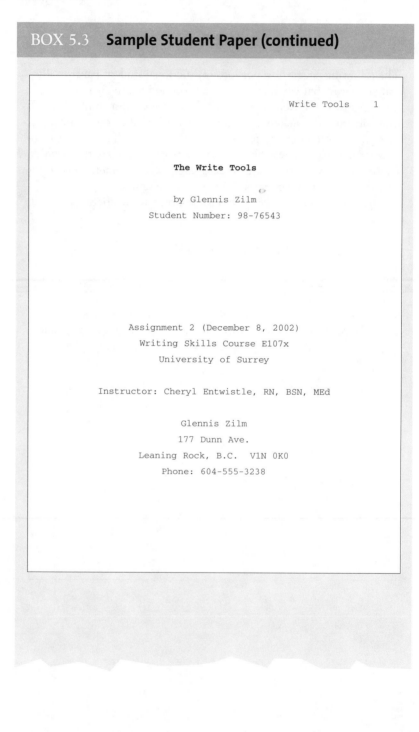

Write Tools   1

The Write Tools

by Glennis Zilm
Student Number: 98-76543

Assignment 2 (December 8, 2002)
Writing Skills Course E107x
University of Surrey

Instructor: Cheryl Entwistle, RN, BSN, MEd

Glennis Zilm
177 Dunn Ave.
Leaning Rock, B.C.   V1N 0K0
Phone: 604-555-3238

BOX 5.3   Sample Student Paper (continued)

Write Tools   2

Table of Contents

BOX 5.3   Sample Student Paper (continued)

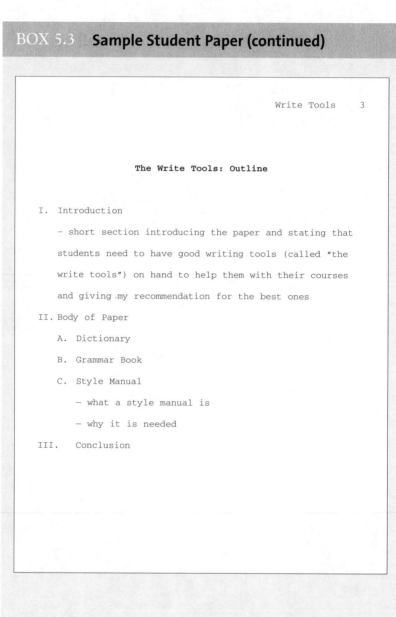

Write Tools   3

The Write Tools: Outline

I. Introduction

    – short section introducing the paper and stating that
    students need to have good writing tools (called "the
    write tools") on hand to help them with their courses
    and giving .my recommendation for the best ones

II. Body of Paper

    A. Dictionary

    B. Grammar Book

    C. Style Manual

        — what a style manual is

        — why it is needed

III.   Conclusion

BOX 5.3   Sample Student Paper (continued)

The Write Tools

Students who hope to do well in their courses need good writing skills. Good writers usually have a shelf of "writing tools" to help them. In particular, students should have three "write tools" on their desks (or on a shelf near the desk): a good dictionary, a basic grammar book, and an approved style manual. In this paper, I give a brief outline of each of these tools and why each is useful. I also recommend the ones I believe students should own.

Dictionary

A good, college-level dictionary is an essential tool for any student writer — even if he or she uses a computer that has a spell checker built in. Dictionaries are much more than lists of words spelled correctly.

BOX 5.3   Sample Student Paper (continued)

They provide information on shades of meaning of synonyms (e.g., character, personality, individuality). They offer information on pronunciation of words (e.g., various pronunciations of *lever*). They point out distinctions in homographs, which are words that sound the same but have different spellings and different meanings (e.g., *root*, *route*) and homonyms, which are words that are spelled and sound the same but have different meanings (e.g., *rose* [flower], *rose* [past tense of *rise*]). They distinguish between various tones of meaning (e.g., formal, informal, slang, derogatory, archaic). They provide valuable information on how a word is used (e.g., as a noun or verb or both). They may even provide information on the origins of a word and the changes it has gone through during its history. As Canadian poet A.M. Klein wrote in 1966: "To know the origins of words is to know the cultural history of mankind" (as cited in Colombo, 1974, p. 313).

BOX 5.3   Sample Student Paper (continued)

Write Tools   6

Dictionaries often reflect the country of origin, such as those written and published in Britain or in the United States. Canadian students should own a Canadian dictionary; the *Gage Canadian Dictionary* (de Wolf, Gregg, Harris, & Scargill, 1997) is my personal choice. It was compiled by a group of distinguished Canadian lexicographers and has been revised and brought up to date to reflect current Canadian usage. The 1983 edition (Avis, Drysdale, Gregg, Neufeldt, & Scargill, 1983) contains a wonderful essay on "Canadian English" originally written in 1967 by Professor Walter S. Avis, one of the original compilers and an expert on Canadian expression; this essay makes one proud of the depth and breadth of the Canadian language. As Avis (1983) wrote:

> The part of Canadian English which is neither British nor American is best illustrated by the vocabulary, for there are hundreds of words which are native to Canada or which have meaning peculiar

BOX 5.3   Sample Student Paper (continued)

Write Tools   7

to Canada.... Few of these words, which may be
called Canadianisms, find their way into British
or American dictionaries, a fact which should
occasion no surprise. (p. xii)

Many courses require that a student writer use a
specific dictionary, such as *Merriam-Webster's
Collegiate Dictionary* (10th ed.) (1999), which is the
latest edition of the dictionary recommended for use by
the American Psychological Association (2001).

Grammar Book

Even students who feel reasonably secure about
their writing skills will benefit by having a sound
grammar reference book among their Write Tools.....

BOX 5.3   Sample Student Paper (continued)

Write Tools   10

References and Bibliography

American Psychological Association. (2001). *Publication*
        manual of the American Psychological Association (5th
        ed.). Washington, DC: Author.
Avis, W. S. (1983). Canadian English. In W. S. Avis, P. D.
        Drysdale, R. J. Gregg, V. E. Neufeldt, & M. H.
        Scargill (Compilers), *Gage Canadian dictionary*
        (pp. xi-xiii). Toronto: Gage.
Avis, W. S., Drysdale, P. D., Gregg, R. J., Neufeldt, V. E.,
        & Scargill, M. H. (Compilers). (1983). *Gage Canadian*
        dictionary. Toronto: Gage.
Buckley, J. (1998). *Fit to print: The Canadian student's*
        guide to essay writing (4th ed.). Toronto: Harcourt
        Brace Canada.
Colombo, J. R. (1974). *Colombo's Canadian quotations*.
        Edmonton: Hurtig.

BOX 5.3   Sample Student Paper (continued)

Day, R. A. (1993). *How to write and publish a scientific paper* (4th ed.). Phoenix, AZ: Oryx Press.

de Wolf, G. D., Gregg, R. J., Harris, B. P., & Scargill, M. H. (Compilers). (1997). *Gage Canadian dictionary* (Rev. ed.). Toronto: Gage.

Entwistle, C. (2002). *E107x Course Syllabus, University of Surrey Department of English*. Surrey, BC: University of Surrey Department of English.

Merriam-Webster's Collegiate Dictionary (10th ed.) (1999). Springfield, MA: Merriam-Webster.

Northey, M., & Timney, B. (1995). *Making sense in psychology and the life sciences: A student's guide to writing and style*. Toronto: Oxford University Press.

An abstract differs from an introduction; even if you write an abstract you still need an introduction to the body of your paper, although the two are similar in content. A main difference is that an abstract usually includes a summary of the findings, whereas an introduction indicates the flow of the article and does not necessarily reveal the findings. Students usually find it best to write the abstract after the body of the paper is in its final draft.

For theses and dissertations, a special and longer abstract is often done. It may be written before the writer begins the research, and it outlines what the graduate candidate proposes to do. The abstract for the final copy of the thesis or dissertation usually is restricted to 350 words, maximum, so that it can be included in one of the indexes of abstracts.

Other kinds of abstracts are submitted to review committees by individuals (including students) who want to give an oral presentation or a poster display at a conference; these abstracts are intended to tell the committee, and later the delegates to the conference, what the writer is prepared to talk about or display. These, too, are often written before the presentation or poster display is prepared.

BODY OF THE PAPER: FORMAT

In Box 5.3, the Sample Student Paper, we show the opening pages of the body of a short paper — a paper that probably would be about 1,000 to 1,200 words long. You will note that there is a brief, one-paragraph introduction. The introduction indicates that the paper is divided into three sections, and then each section opens with a heading. If you look back at the table of contents and outline for this paper, you will see that only two levels of heading are needed: the title, which is repeated (as per APA style) at the top centre of the opening page of the body of the paper; and one level of subheading.

Our Sample Student Paper shows some differences from the style recommended for articles in the APA (2001) *Manual*; however, it is consistent with the advice that the *Manual* gives in the section that discusses student papers. In the section on student papers, the *Manual* makes it clear that student papers — because they are "final" copies — may differ from "copy" manuscripts being prepared to send to editors of APA journals (p. 321). So, unless your instructor has provided specific guidelines telling you otherwise, you may wish to follow our guidelines and use bold face for titles, underlining subheadings, which are at the left margin, italics for book and journal titles, and extra spaces before subheadings, among other minor style changes. In fact, you may even wish to single-space long quotations (which we do not do) and single-space tables (which we did not show in the example, but which we would recommend).

We put subheads at the left margin and underlined them; we could have chosen to place them in the centre or to use bold typeface. (See Box 5.2 to review the information on subheadings.)

You also can see on these opening pages the two methods of formatting quotations within the body of the paper. The APA (2001) *Manual* advises that if the quotation is less than 40 words, it should be included within the text paragraph; if longer, the quotation is indented (use the indent key) 5 to 7 spaces (same spacing as the tab indent used for the paragraph) from the left margin. Note that the indented quotation is *not* enclosed in quotation marks. Look the sample paper over carefully; you may find many other small points that will be helpful to you as you format your own paper.

REFERENCES AND BIBLIOGRAPHY

The "References and Bibliography" page of the Sample Student Paper in Box 5.3 shows only a few of the references that might be included if the paper were complete, but the ones included are enough to give you some ideas and start you thinking about the formatting of this page. Because this was a short paper (up to 1,500 words), the references and bibliography are combined, not presented separately; thus there are a couple of books in the list that were not referred to in the paper.

Note that the References list always starts on a new page (because it is a separate section and not part of the main text or body), but that the subhead is in the same style as the subheadings in the main body of the paper (in this example, underlined and at the left margin). You might also wish to notice how the listing appeared in this section for the A. M. Klein quotation (taken from a secondary source).

CHECKLIST FOR FINAL TYPING OF STUDENT PAPERS (APA STYLE)

The following checklist reviews some of the points you need to keep in mind when shining up your paper.

- Use white copy paper, size 8.5" x 11".
- Set at least one-inch margins at top, bottom, and left and right sides of all pages.
- Justify the left margin, but leave the right margin unjustified ("ragged").
- Use a standard 12-point typeface with serifs, such as Times Roman, CG Times, Courier, or Pica.
- Double-space lines in the main text (and in most other parts of the paper *unless* other spacings would improve appearance and readability).

- Number all pages in the top right-hand corner beginning with the title page.
- Identify your running head on the cover page and set it to appear on each page of your paper either five spaces to the left of the page number or immediately above the page number.
- Read the paper aloud: is it easy to read, or do you stumble anywhere?
- Check the length of your sentences: are there too many long sentences?
- Do too many sentences start the same way? Look especially for sentences with weak openings such as "There are ..." or "This is ..." or "It was ...."
- Check for improper use of first-person pronouns (*I, we, my, our, me, ours*).
- Have you used jargon, slang, or clichés?
- Are too many sentences in the passive voice?
- Check the style of your title, headings, and subheadings.
- Check the spelling of any word about which you are not completely certain; if you use a computer and have a spell checker, learn how to use it.
- Check the use of capitals: are they consistent? Do you have a reason for using the capital letters you used throughout your paper?
- Check the punctuation: have you used a comma before the word *and* in a series of three or more items? Do you have too many commas? Are there quotation marks where they are needed? Have you used apostrophes appropriately? Are there too many dashes and exclamation points (which signal an informal tone)?
- Proofread the finished, printed copy through a final time; do not change your content, but make any minor corrections neatly in black ink on the final version.
- Keep a copy of your paper; even the best instructors occasionally misplace a paper.
- Always remember that your instructor's requirements outrank all other style guidelines.
- Think SMART.

Submitting the Paper

Finally, you are ready to submit your paper. Most instructors prefer to get the paper without an envelope or cover; some prefer an envelope, especially if the paper is to be returned by mail, or a cover to help keep papers separate from one another during marking. APA guidelines advise that you submit the paper with a paperclip in the top left corner, rather than stapled; this makes it easier for both editors and instructors, who sometimes like to spread the paper out and look at various pages at the same time (e.g., the body of the paper and the references).

Try to submit the paper on time, unless you have a good reason for a delay. If you need an extension, ask for one rather than just submitting the paper late.

Summary

This chapter has concentrated on the final rungs of the writing PROCESS ladder: the formatting and typing up of the final drafts and the layout of a student paper. Please do not be overwhelmed by what seem to be so many rules; soon they will come almost automatically. During your student days you may write 50 or more papers, so learning the rules early will pay off in the long run.

We want to stress that you should think SMART in every written communication and consider the stages of the writing PROCESS. After reading this far in the book, you should be much more informed than when you started and have a better idea of your strengths and weaknesses. You should realize that you need good resources and tools to assist you as you write. You will need to work hard on the message of each new paper; most of that content will come from the courses you take and the readings and materials assigned for them, but you will also have improved your ability to find new information on your own. You should be aware of the importance of your audience (your instructor or, sometimes, a designated marker). Students who ask questions and discuss the feedback given with the paper usually are much more successful than those who do not. You should now have a good understanding of the route (the student paper), which, though it does have many rules, also has maps (style guides). And you should now understand how tone affects your writing and realize that student papers are relatively formal.

Writing is hard work, and probably always will be — but so are many other enjoyable activities, such as gardening, mountain climbing, or hockey. Look on this learning experience as a challenge that will pay off and make your future more enjoyable. The writing skills that you practise now will benefit you later in your nursing career.

Exercises

Two self-assessment exercises that review points to look for in the shining-up step are included here. Try them.

EXERCISE 5.1   **Grammar, Usage, Spelling, and Punctuation**

This short paragraph contains errors in grammar, usage, spelling, and punctuation. See how many you can spot and correct.

> In order to efficiently apply for most senior positions, resumes should be used. Potential applicants often seek advise from communication experts in designing their résumés, however some of the suggestions from these consultants are a bit flamboyant and they are unsuited to conservative health care institutions. All recommendations should be weighed carefully. Noone should accept poor council which may effect their futures.

COMMENTS ON EXERCISE 5.1   **Grammar, Usage, Spelling, and Punctuation**

1. Change *In order to efficiently apply* to *To apply* (unnecessary words).
2. Delete *most* (unnecessary).
3. Change *resumes* to *résumés* (check spelling and Canadian usage in *Gage Canadian Dictionary* [de Wolf, Gregg, Harris, & Scargill, 1997] and be consistent throughout the paper; note that the spelling in the next sentence is *résumés*).
4. Change *résumés should be used* to *applicants should use résumés* (résumés do not apply for senior positions — applicants do; poor sentence and passive voice).
5. Change *Potential applicants* to *Many job hunters* (clarity; shorter words; prevents repetition of applicants in the rewritten version).
6. Change *advise* to *advice* (either a misused word or a typing error).
7. Change *in designing their résumés* to *about résumé design* (ambiguous pronoun reference; *their* could refer to experts or to applicants).
8. Change the comma to a semicolon before *however* and insert a comma after *however* (original is a "run-on sentence"; alternative: change the comma to a period and start the next sentence with *However* and a comma).
9. Delete *of the* (unnecessary).
10. Change *consultents* to *consultants* (either a spelling mistake or a typing error; tighten the sentence by removing *a bit*, a lazy and vague modifier, then reword latter part of sentence both to remove the pronoun *they*, which could refer to *consultants*, and to reduce the length of the sentence).
11. Change *All recommendations should be weighed carefully* to *Weigh recommendations carefully* (removes passive voice).

12. Change *Noone* to *No one* (either a spelling mistake or a typing error).
13. Change *council* to *counsel* (misuse of word).
14. Change *which* to *that* (misuse of word).
15. Change *effect* to *affect* (misuse of word).
16. Change *their futures* to *his or her future* (lack of agreement; pronoun[s] must agree in number with *No one*; alternative: change *their futures* to *one's future*).

The following is the revised, polished version (48 words compared with 62 words in original; average number of words per sentence 12 compared with 15.5 in original; one long sentence with 23 words compared with one long sentence with 33 words in original):

> To apply for senior positions, applicants should use résumés. Many job hunters seek advice from communication experts about résumé design; however, suggestions from some consultants may be unsuitable for health care professionals. Weigh recommendations carefully. No one should accept poor counsel that may affect his or her future.

EXERCISE 5.2   Shining Up the Final Copy

The following exercise reviews the kind of shining up you should do in your final review.

1. Delete extraneous words in the following sentences.
   - He is in the process of drawing up the nominations.
   - She intends to take action without further delay.
2. Polish the following poor sentences.
   - She did not think that it was unimportant to wear neat, professional dress.
   - The union was not unwilling to negotiate on the offer.
   - Well Known Hospital (WKH) will be responsible for the development and execution of a health promotion day designed to increase awareness in the local community about WKH's Wellness Clinic.
3. Think about the double meanings in the following sentences.
   - Yesterday, the police tied the suspect to the car used in the holdup.
   - New mothers find it much harder to manage when they have children.

COMMENTS ON EXERCISE 5.2   **Shining Up the Final Copy**

1. Following are shorter, clearer versions.
   - He is drawing up the nominations.
   - She intends to take action now.

2. The following are improved versions.
   - She thought that neat professional dress was important. (This version avoids double negatives.)
   - The union was willing to negotiate on the offer.
   - Well Known Hospital will develop and carry out a health promotion day to inform the local community about its Wellness Clinic.
     OR
   - Well Known Hospital will develop and carry out a health promotion day to help make the local community aware of its Wellness Clinic.

3. You could rewrite these sentences several ways, if you have time. The two humorous examples should remind you that sometimes you get too close to your work — although a sentence makes good sense to you, it may not make good sense to your readers.

CHAPTER SIX

SMART Ways for Other Routes in Nursing

The SMART elements of communication and the steps in the writing PROCESS will work for you throughout your career. Once you have practised using them and have learned the basics related to each type of written communication, you should be able to master each new route fairly quickly. In this chapter, we go over the fundamentals of a variety of routes — business letters, memos, e-mail messages, résumés, reports, and articles — that you will meet in your career. Each one requires practice, of course, and you can learn and apply numerous details for each type of communication; in fact, there is at least one book devoted to each of the routes described in this chapter. But if you think SMART and draw on the basics from earlier in this book, you should adapt well to all routes.

BUSINESS LETTERS

You learned the fundamentals of business letters in grade school and have probably already had to write a number of business letters. For example, many schools of nursing require that you write a formal letter of application, which is one type of business letter. During your course, you may also need to communicate formally with your school of nursing or with an instructor, and you may need to use a business letter to do that.

All letters have much the same basic form. As the writer of the letter, you are the source. Even if you are sending much the same message (e.g., "I am applying for a job"), each audience (e.g., friend, personnel officer) is likely different. Even if you are a friend of the person to whom you are sending a business letter, you treat it differently because it is not just sent to that person but may become part of the office or agency files. The main differences between a personal letter (i.e., one you would send to a friend) and a business letter apply to a few rules of route and a distinct difference in tone. However, even business letters can have differences in tone, from highly formal to informal but still businesslike.

Almost all business letters are done on stationery that is 8.5" x 11". The paper should be of good quality and be either a basic white or a neutral, formal color (cream, grey, pale blue) and should have business-size envelopes (9" x 4" or 9.5" x 4") that match in color. Letters are folded into three to fit into these envelopes. You can get colored and printed (e.g., floral) stationery in these sizes (mainly because they fit into computer printers easily), but save them for personal letters.

Should a business letter always be typed? You need to think SMART and work out your own answer to that question. For example, when you are just starting out to find employment, you may not have much money, and paying a typist to type letters of application to potential employers can be costly. If you write neatly and legibly, a short, handwritten letter of application that accompanies a typed résumé will probably be acceptable to most hospital or agency personnel offices; some potential employers like to see your handwriting because it often reveals details about you (e.g., whether you can spell). On the other hand, if you are writing an application asking for several thousand dollars of funding for equipment on your unit, then you would be wise to use a well-qualified secretary employed by the agency to do the layout. If you are writing a letter of thanks to the president of the volunteers on behalf of your unit, a legible, handwritten note on hospital stationery would usually be acceptable and might convey a warmer, more friendly tone than a typed letter. If, on behalf of the staff of your unit, you are writing a letter of condolence to the family of a former patient, a handwritten formal note might be the most appropriate format, even though this communication might be classified as a business letter.

BASIC FORMAT OF A BUSINESS LETTER

As you may remember from your school days, the basic format for a business letter is:

- address or letterhead;
- date;
- file numbers (optional);

- inside address (complete name and address of the individual and company to whom you are writing, including all details, such as postal code);
- reference line(s) (optional; may go below the salutation);
- salutation (the "Dear ..." line, sometimes optional);
- body of letter (in which you use the outline discussed in Chapter 2);
- complimentary close;
- signature;
- typed name (sometimes optional; e.g., it would be omitted if you use your own letterhead);
- stenographic reference (writer's initials/typist's initials); and
- note regarding enclosures or copies.

Boxes 6.1 and 6.2 show the basic format for two relatively simple business letters. The first is set in a style known as "flush left," which has been adopted by many businesses in recent years; all new sections of the letter, including paragraphs, start at the left-hand margin. The second letter follows a more traditional indented style and is suitable for handwritten business letters. If you have access to the services of a typist or typing pool, you can usually leave the decisions about layout of the business letter to the typist. If you type your own business letters, follow the flush left style, because it is by far the easiest to set up. Instructors at secretarial schools teach rules about setting up the spacing between the various sections, but if you have to do the spacing yourself, then position the letter in the centre of the page and leave double spaces between sections. Some of these basic parts deserve a few additional comments — especially because some of the comments apply to other routes, such as memos and e-mail messages.

ADDRESS OR LETTERHEAD

If you are writing a business letter on behalf of your employer, you would use the letterhead of the hospital, agency, or company; you are acting as a source on behalf of that agency. The letterhead contains the return address, and all mail in reply to your letter would be sent to that address. You may need to add a typed line immediately below to indicate how mail should be directed to you within the agency (e.g., the name of the ward).

You would almost never use a company letterhead and ask for a reply to be sent to you at another address (e.g., your home address), although there are a few exceptions (e.g., when you write on behalf of a club or association and wish to speed up mail delivery); you need, however, to make this point clearly in the body of the letter.

BOX 6.1   Sample Business Letter, Flush Left Style

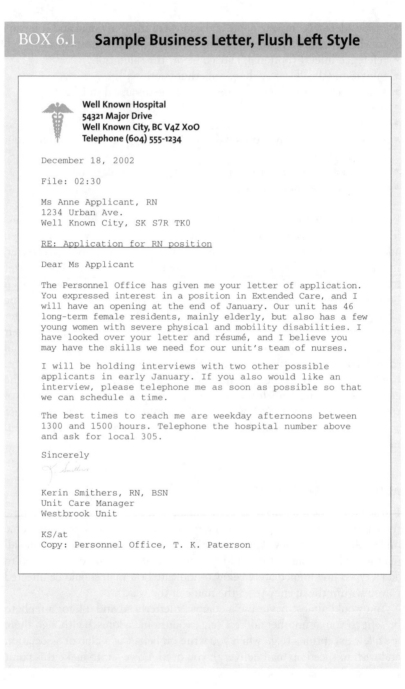

Well Known Hospital
54321 Major Drive
Well Known City, BC V4Z X0O
Telephone (604) 555-1234

December 18, 2002

File: 02:30

Ms Anne Applicant, RN
1234 Urban Ave.
Well Known City, SK S7R TK0

RE: Application for RN position

Dear Ms Applicant

The Personnel Office has given me your letter of application. You expressed interest in a position in Extended Care, and I will have an opening at the end of January. Our unit has 46 long-term female residents, mainly elderly, but also has a few young women with severe physical and mobility disabilities. I have looked over your letter and résumé, and I believe you may have the skills we need for our unit's team of nurses.

I will be holding interviews with two other possible applicants in early January. If you also would like an interview, please telephone me as soon as possible so that we can schedule a time.

The best times to reach me are weekday afternoons between 1300 and 1500 hours. Telephone the hospital number above and ask for local 305.

Sincerely

Kerin Smithers, RN, BSN
Unit Care Manager
Westbrook Unit

KS/at
Copy: Personnel Office, T. K. Paterson

BOX 6.2   Sample Business Letter, Indented Style

Well Known Hospital   December 18, 2002
54321 Major Drive
Well Known City, BC V4Z X0O
Telephone (604) 555-1234

Mrs. R. K. Helper, President
 WKH Auxiliary
  c/o 123 Country Ave.
   Well Known Suburb, AB T7K R8O

Dear Mrs. Helper

   On behalf of Westbrook Extended Care Unit, I wish to thank
you for the two new Ezy-Lift chairs donated this month by
the Auxiliary. These two chairs are valuable for assisting
arthritic elderly residents get to their feet with a minimum of nursing assistance. One resident told me this morning how much she likes the chair and how much safer she
feels.

   WKH Auxiliary has done so much for our Hospital, and I
want you to know how much your gifts are appreciated by residents and staff. Please, the next time you are at the hospital, drop by the unit, and I will arrange to show you how
delightfully the chairs fit into the sun porch.

   Please extend our thanks to all members of your group.

                              Sincerely

                              (Ms) Kerin Smithers, RN
                              Unit Care Manager
                              Westbrook Unit

You may also need to write business letters from your home on your own behalf (e.g., to apply for a job, to write to a politician or a newspaper stating an opinion, or to ask for a correction to a bank document). In today's world of computers, you may wish to develop your own letterhead, as shown in Box 6.3. Save your letterhead on a disk or your hard drive so that you can use it whenever you write a business letter. You can also buy a printed letterhead for yourself (expensive) or hire a secretarial service to type up and run off a few dozen copies for you to use (much less expensive). Such letterheads are not difficult to design, but you do need to keep a few SMART principles in mind as you do so. For business, the letterhead should be slightly formal; plain is generally better than fancy — but you can think SMART. For example, Madonna might select a more daring letterhead if she were writing to a producer to line up a job than you would choose if you were writing to a public health department asking for a staff position. If you (source) weigh the message, audience, and tone, you should be able to design a personal business letterhead that is creative and suitable.

INFORMATION BEFORE THE BODY OF THE LETTER

Many people wonder whether they should write December 22, 2002 or 22 December 2002 or some other version for the date of the letter. We like the former, with the month spelled out, but you can use the format you want. You might want to note that health care agencies tend to use the international format (the latter version).

A file number is only necessary in a large agency, such as a hospital, and you have to learn the method used. A file number might be used on job applications, as in the sample letter shown in Box 6.1. If you are responding to a letter that used a file number, you should quote that number in any further correspondence. For example, if Anne Applicant responded to Kerin Smithers, she would put in this line:

Your file number: 02:30

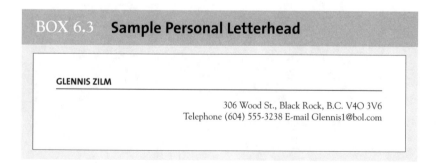

BOX 6.3   **Sample Personal Letterhead**

GLENNIS ZILM

306 Wood St., Black Rock, B.C. V4O 3V6
Telephone (604) 555-3238 E-mail Glennis1@bol.com

The inside address is an essential part of a business letter and should be as complete as possible. For best results, you should always attempt to find out the name of a person to whom to address your letter (although this information is not always available). For example, if you are writing a letter to the editor of a professional journal, you should check a recent copy of the journal and find out the name of the editor. If you are sending a job application to a small hospital or agency in your area, you may want to telephone the switchboard and ask to whom the letter should be addressed; you may not want to do this if it involves a costly long distance call. If you are writing to a large urban hospital, where there are likely several people working in the department, you could address the letter to the Personnel Office or the Human Resources Department. Remember, however, that almost any reader likes to be addressed by name.

Using a name for the inside address is also helpful in writing the salutation; you then address the individual by name. Thus, you do not have to use the completely out of date "To Whom It May Concern" or the old-fashioned "Dear Sir or Madam"; some recipients find these salutations (especially the latter) offensive. Many letter writers worry about how to write the salutation when they have only the initials of the person or have a first name for a woman but do not know whether to write "Ms.," "Mrs.," or "Miss." Our advice to these worriers is to concentrate on writing a good message in the body of the letter. Then simply think SMART about the details of the salutation. If you do find out the name, also try to find out if it belongs to a Mrs. or Miss or Dr. You can also use the first name or initials with the last name if that is the way the person has signed a letter to you (e.g., "Dear Mary Jones" or "Dear M.T. Jones"). If you do not have a name, you can omit the salutation altogether and just use a reference line. (See sample letter of application for a job in Box 6.4.)

The reference line usually highlights the subject of the letter (as in the example in Box 6.1). You can use "RE:" or "Re:" or "Subject:". The reference line is usually underlined, but some sources prefer to use all capital letters. A reference line might also be used to highlight something important, such as "Personal and confidential."

Some style guides for business letters say that you can use the reference line to bring the letter to the attention of some person within the company, as in the following example.

Personnel Office
Well Known Hospital
54321 Major Drive
Well Known City, BC V4Z X0O

ATTENTION: Mary Jones, Personnel Officer

Dear Ms. Jones

BOX 6.4   Sample Job Application Letter

```
1234 Urban Street
Thunder Bay, AB T8G 0X0

June 23, 2001

Human Resources/Personnel Office
Well Known Regional Hospital
4321 Main Street
Prince George, BC V2L 0N0

RE: Application for Registered Nurse Position

   My husband and I are moving to Prince George in mid-
August, and I am seeking a position as a staff nurse. He
will be joining the teaching staff at Prince George
Elementary School.
   As you will see from my résumé, I graduated in late
April from the School of Nursing at Thunder Bay Community
College, and I have passed my Registered Nurse exams. I am
registered with the Alberta Association of Registered
Nurses, and I applied for registration with the Registered
Nurses Association of B.C. earlier this month.
   Since graduation, I have been working as a casual relief
nurse at the Eagle Ridge Hospital near Thunder Bay, mainly
in the Long Term Care Units. The local hospitals do not
have any openings for full-time staff, but I have been
assured that my work skills are excellent, and I would be
in line for a full-time position should one arise. My unit
supervisors have agreed to supply letters if you require
references. As well as my nursing jobs, I have worked part
time as an assistant in a day care centre (12 infants).
   I would like to receive information about your hospital
and application forms for a possible RN position. If you
expect to have an opening before mid-August and would like
to discuss it with me, I can be reached by telephone at
(403) 555-2112.

Sincerely

(Mrs.) Geraldine Summers, RN
```

Points to note

This preliminary letter, sent before a move to a new location, should elicit application forms and some information about the hospital and its human relations department (perhaps including the name of the person who receives the applications for RN positions).

This kind of address might be used if you had spoken to Mary Jones on the telephone before you sent the letter but wanted it to convey the message that you were not writing to her personally but sending a general letter of application.

INFORMATION AFTER THE BODY OF THE LETTER

The complimentary close comes immediately after the body of the letter, separated by a double space. The complimentary close most commonly used now in business letters is "Sincerely," although some companies use "Yours truly." Some complimentary closings are long outdated, such as "Your faithful servant." (And, after reading Chapter 3 in this book, you would never use "Very truly yours," would you?) If you have had a long business correspondence with a person or have come to know him or her, you might want to alter the closing for that person and use something like "Best wishes."

After the complimentary close, you leave some space for your signature. For business letters to someone you do not know, you should generally avoid using nicknames or diminutives and develop a consistent signature (e.g., Marjorie Jones rather than Marj Jones). Once you know the correspondent well, you may elect to sign with the name that she or he calls you (e.g., Marj). You do not write in your courtesy title (e.g., Mrs.), your degree(s) (e.g., RN), or your title (e.g., Unit Manager).

The typed signature line goes below your signature — even if the latter is legible. This line does contain the courtesy title, degree(s), and title; you may need an extra line if your job title is long. Make it clear in the typed signature how you wish to be addressed. For example, you may sign the letter "Nancy Nadon," but the typed signature might read "(Mrs.) Nancy Nadon, R.N." or "Nancy Nadon, RN (Miss)."

If you type your own letter, you do not need a stenographic reference. If a secretary types the letter, he or she will put in your initials followed by his or her own.

If you are adding enclosures to the letter or sending a copy of the letter to some other person or department, make a note to this effect by adding the accepted abbreviations for enclosure (enc) or carbon copy (cc).

HELPFUL HINTS FOR THE BODY OF THE LETTER

Although we have taken a number of pages to go over the rules of the route for letters, always remember that the message in the body of the letter is the most important part. The ways to develop a good body of a letter are the same as those already described in Chapters 1 through 5. First of all, think SMART.

Keep in mind who you (source) are and why you are writing. If you are writing on behalf of your employer, be aware that what you say and how you say it will reflect on your employer (and ultimately on your job). Sometimes (as in the example of the letter to the president of WKH Auxiliary) you are writing on behalf of those who work for you.

Work out what your message really is; you may even want to summarize it in the reference line so that it will be at the top of the letter. Your message should be presented in the same three-part outline that works for assignments. The opening paragraph, which should be short, is the introduction and tells the recipient what the letter is about. The body of the message is conveyed in the next paragraph or two (or more, if necessary). The final paragraph, which also should be short, is the conclusion and should sum up what you want the recipient of the letter to do. Like the conclusion to a student paper, the final paragraph or sentence will stay in the reader's mind, so it should be positive, interesting, stimulating, and creative. Depending on the importance of the letter, you may want to spend extra time on the beginning and ending as well as on the important basic information in the middle. If you are writing a letter to your mother, she will likely be so delighted to hear from you that you can open with a trite remark such as "How are you? I am fine" and close with "Give my love to dad, and ask him to send me an extra five dollars for a pizza." On the other hand, if you are writing a letter to all the graduates of your school of nursing to raise funds for a student scholarship, you should be particularly creative so that all the graduates will read the opening, and the body, and the conclusion — and then send some money!

Try to visualize the person to whom you are writing (audience) and even think about the setting in which he or she will be reading your letter (e.g., a busy office, with 17 other similar letters on the desk). Think about the information your reader will want, and try to present your message with consideration for the reader's point of view. What information does this person want or need in your letter?

The rules of the route for the business letter have been covered above. Adapt them to meet your needs (as source) as well as the needs of the message and the audience.

Finally, consider the tone of the letter. Try to see, again in your mind's eye, the recipient of your letter as a friend (even if you are writing a letter to complain about something). This visualization exercise will usually help you to set a good tone, and you can choose words that will make a positive impression. Is your business letter to be a begging letter, a demanding letter, a whining letter, a bitter letter? Even if the message is negative, you can use a positive tone; the reactions of your audience are likely to lead to better results. For example, if you are writing to complain about a mistake, the individual who gets the letter is probably not the one who made the mistake; why antagonize this person? If you get the reader on your side, the mistake is more likely to be corrected.

After thinking SMART, go over the steps of the writing PROCESS: Plan * Research * Organize * Create * Edit * Shine * Send! Just as with an assignment, if you take a few minutes to plan, research, and organize before you start to write your letter, you will write more like a pro. The letter is more likely to do what you want it to do. Of course, you should not spend hours or days on every simple letter. But the more important the letter, the more important it is to take time to plan, research, and organize so that the letter will be effective.

Think about letters of application for a job, for example. Suppose you write several letters quickly (without taking time to plan, research, organize, create, edit, and shine them before you submit them). You have wasted time and effort if those letters do not result in job interviews. Once you have done all the work for one letter, the next ones can almost be copied with only a little time needed to think SMART (e.g., Is this the same type of audience? Are the same skills required?). You may want to create a file of good letters that you can use as models. Many senior nurse managers do this.

Other examples of letters that nurses might find helpful can be found later in this chapter. Look these over for ideas as well.

Keep your letter as short as possible. Business people usually read one-page letters as soon as they open them; they put longer letters (especially those of more than two pages) into the in-basket to read when they have more time (which is almost never!).

MEMOS

Memos are a vital part of a business environment, and if you are working in a hospital or other health care agency, you will likely have to write memos as part of your job. You therefore need to understand the rules of this route. Fortunately, many of the rules are similar to those for letters. In fact, memos are really just shorter, less formal letters done on a different type of stationery. For formal memos in some agencies, you may need to use all the parts of a business letter, including file numbers. On the other hand, some short, handwritten memos are merely notes between two friends or colleagues confirming a time for lunch. Thinking SMART will help you.

The basic format for a memo is shown in Box 6.5. Note that the essential items in a memo are:

- date;
- receiver's identity and department;
- sender's identity and departmental address and phone number;
- subject statement; and
- message (finishing with recommendations for follow-up).

The optional items in a memo include

- signature;
- copies (sometimes there is a section marked "Copies To:");
- enclosures or attachments;
- stenographic reference;
- file numbers; and
- security classification (in agencies where documents must be kept confidential).

Memo forms are often only 8.5" x 5.5", which should give you a clue about length. Keep your memos short, and usually keep them to one subject; it is often more efficient for your readers (always consider the audience) if you send two memos when you have two subjects. Doing so may not seem more convenient for you (source), but if the receiver can jot a short note in reply at the bottom of a memo and return it to you immediately, then you will get the action you want more quickly.

Some agencies have supplies of "round trip memo forms," which allow you to write the original and one or two copies; they are used when you must keep a file related to that memo, such as might be required if you are sending a memo seeking action on a drug error or reporting a patient's fall. You keep the bottom copy for your records (e.g., perhaps attached to the patient's chart) and send the top copies. The receiver writes a reply for you at the bottom of the page, keeps the bottom copy for her or his files, and returns the original. These memos are often useful when you must send copies to keep others informed.

In some agencies, memos are intended to be posted on a bulletin board or filed in a binder so that all staff can see them. If so, you now have a new audience for your memo — and this readership should affect how you write the message. If the memo is to be posted, would it be more effective set up as a posterlike announcement? For example, if you are announcing the time and place of the unit's July 1 picnic, perhaps flyers on flag-laden colored stationery prepared expressly for bulletin boards would be more effective than a memo. On the other hand, a poster would not be appropriate for a hospital policy directive that needs to reach all staff.

If the memo is to be filed in a binder on the unit, then you may want to consider how to make your memo more useful; for example, perhaps you

BOX 6.5   Sample Memo

Well Known Hospital
54321 Major Drive
Well Known City, BC V4Z X0O
Telephone (604) 555-1234

INTERDEPARTMENTAL MEMO

TO: _Mary Winters, Unit Manager OR_   DATE: _14/12/2002_

FROM: _Dee Stanos, Staff Library Volunteer_   PHONE: _(250) 555-1234_

SUBJECT: _Article on Latex Allergies_

You spoke to me some time ago about articles on latex allergies. Have you seen the following?

Latex Allergy Update: Clinical Practice and Unresolved Issues, by E. Meeropol. *WOCN: Journal of Wound, Ostomy and Continence Nursing*, Vol. 23, No. 4, July 1996.

This journal was recently donated to the library and has been placed on the "new reading" shelves. The article says those who have latex allergies often react as well when they eat certain foods, including bananas, avocados, and foods sterilized with ethylene oxide.

If you would like me to make a photocopy for you, please leave a message on my answering machine at home and I will do so the next time I am in the hospital.

---

should use 8.5" x 11" paper (rather than the shorter form) and ensure that holes are punched in the paper before it is sent. Sometimes it is more effective if the memo is circulated within a department rather than posted; if you believe that circulation would be the most efficient method and would make your message more useful, then you should attach a circulation list to the memo rather than expect the receiver to do that. Remember that each of the SMART elements interacts with and influences the others.

As you become more senior in your job, your attitude to and use of memos may change. Most staff nurses who attended our workshops reported that they resented memos, perhaps because many management memos seem to come across as "Now hear this" directives. Managers tend to write this way because they have a responsibility to communicate, and "Do this" memos usually seem quick and effective. When you join the management team, however, you can take action to reduce the negative impact that this type of memo seems to have on staff. For example, when you become a head nurse or unit manager, you can try to send fewer memos and have more face-to-face meetings with staff. You can set up headline cards (e.g., "New Directives from Pharmacy") and then post all policy memos from pharmacy in that section of the bulletin board. Or you may choose to file them in special binders in which staff can review them. You can review incoming memos yourself and use a highlighter to emphasize relevant points for your staff. These hints, however, relate more to management techniques than to writing skills.

The important point is to think SMART when it comes to writing memos. If you make them short, simple, clear, interesting, friendly, appropriate, and easy for the receiver to handle, your memos will be effective.

E-MAIL MESSAGES

Within many hospitals and agencies, e-mail messages and other forms of electronic communication (e.g., scheduling of meetings) have replaced many of the telephone calls, short, informal memos, and business letters that were so common in the past. E-mail messages are a special form of written communication, and the SMART elements apply. Messages to communicate with friends are likely informal, perhaps with contractions and added "smilies," such as ;-) (a wink) or :-((a frown). Business messages, including communications with your instructors, may need a more formal tone (see also Chapter 1), and business e-mail memos and letters are often strictly formal, written in professional language, and perhaps sent as attached files so that the format is also formal.

Within agencies, e-mail is used because it is quicker than interdepartmental mail and less intrusive than telephone calls. Between agencies, it is often used because it is cheaper than long distance telephone calls and faster than regular post office delivery ("snail mail").

Most e-mail messages should be relatively short. If a message is longer than can be read on a single screen, the receiver will have to scroll through it or print it out. Either is time-consuming, so keep your e-mail message to the point.

The format for e-mail documents is often determined by the software programs used or by the telecommunications system that supplies the online service. Most formats are similar to a Memo page. The program usually has a "From:" line identifying the sender (although often by a code name), a "Date:" line, a "To:" line that gives the receiver's e-mail address, and a "Subject:" line in which you describe *briefly* what the message will be about.

Remember, too, that there are concerns about e-mail messages; for example, they can carry computer viruses. As well, many busy people receive numerous business e-mails in a day, and they appreciate it if you keep them short and businesslike. (Consider your audience.) Many receivers may also be concerned about junk mail, confidentiality, and privacy. Some receivers delete e-mail messages unread if they appear frivolous or unimportant, so be certain you describe the contents appropriately in the subject line if you are sending a message to someone who does not know you by your user name or address.

Not all receivers routinely print out their messages, so you also need to be aware that your message may not be kept. Some e-mail systems allow the receiver to create folders or files in which to store messages, but not all do. Most programs also delete mail automatically after a specific period of time, so if your recipient is away (e.g., on holidays or a business trip), your e-mail may disappear.

You can also send your message to several receivers all at the same time (through the copy or group-send method); this is a wonderful way to deal with some items you want to send to a specific group (e.g., announcements of meetings, agendas, minutes). You can also "Forward" messages to others simply at the click of an icon. Remember to limit copies and forwarded mail to only those who need the information, however, or you may gain a reputation as someone who sends junk mail.

Most e-mail programs allow the receiver to "Reply" simply at the press of an icon on the screen, and busy people like to use this option. This is another reason why you should keep your message short and limit it to one topic.

If you use a computer often, you will no doubt be familiar with the emotional conversational styles (tone) that can be conveyed through typing. For example, use of all CAPITAL LETTERS is generally considered "shouting." You will often see typing errors and many of the common errors in informal e-mail messages — but why waste time and energy if the point of your message is to ask someone if she is ready to go for lunch?

You can also send business letters by e-mail, especially when you are anxious to have the message arrive quickly. In such cases, we suggest that, after you have filled in the opening lines of the e-mail, you should format the e-mail exactly as you would a business letter on a page. You can use a simple letterhead with your name, address, phone number, and e-mail address at the top of the page, then the date and inside address, and then a line that says

Letter sent by e-mail

just before the salutation.

You may also choose to send this kind of important business letter by a file transfer. In this case, you would set up the letter in your word-processing program, following all the rules for the format of a business letter, and then save it, giving it a file name. You would then send the file attached to a brief e-mail message. In the e-mail message you should, however, say something like: "Letter attached as file named < :\gzletter.wpd > ; this alerts the receiver to notice that there is a file attached, and its name, so that he or she can easily retrieve it later from the document files in the computer. If the letter is vital, you may want to send a hard copy in the mail as well.

Use the SMART principles. Is the e-mail route suitable for your message? Do you need to transfer printed information quickly? Does the format matter? The basic e-mail format is usually best suited for short messages, although you can attach files or send documents. For example, you can send an assignment or a report via e-mail as an attached file, which can then be printed by the receiver. This method works wonderfully for the exchange of draft documents, but often the formatting is not suitable for finished documents. You also need to consider whether your receiver likes to use e-mail and file transfer — and whether he or she knows how.

RÉSUMÉS

One of the important written communications you will need during your nursing career is a résumé. A résumé (sometimes written without the accents) is a brief summary of educational and employment experiences that is submitted with a job application. In today's world, chances are that you will change jobs during your working lifetime *at least* six times; for many nurses, up to 15 different jobs during their working careers is common. Sometimes these changes are within a single agency, but sometimes you may even decide to change to a different field.

To develop a good résumé and keep it up to date so that you can apply for positions in coming years, consider starting a résumé file for yourself. In it, you can keep all the important background materials that you will need in future years, such as your high school certificate, nursing graduation certificates, registration examination results, copies of official documents pertaining to courses and marks, and information on special courses taken (e.g., CPR certificate). These documents will come in handy for many years and will help you to keep dates correct. (Believe us, you will forget such information!) Start a good file, and keep copies of your résumés in it for future reference.

A résumé may not be so important for that first nursing job after graduation, but it will become more and more important in later years. Hospitals and most other health care agencies generally prefer that applicants for staff nurse positions fill out an application form designed especially for the institution; it makes it easy for a personnel officer to review the information quickly and according to the special needs of the hospital or agency. If that is the case, you must fill out the form — but you can also attach your résumé, which carries additional weight and shows that you know something about job hunting. Furthermore, if you have your résumé on hand when you fill out the application form, you are more likely to have all the information (e.g., dates) you need. So you should develop a résumé, or at least a worksheet that you can follow when filling out applications, soon after graduation.

You can hire other people to help you prepare and type a résumé, but if you learn how to do it yourself, by thinking SMART, you will end up with a much better message. You may need to hire a typist, but the most useful résumé tends to be the one you have prepared yourself.

A résumé is usually your first contact with a potential employer, so, most importantly, you need to weigh the needs of the receiver. Most employers spend less than a minute looking over a résumé when it first arrives, so consider using ways to make yours stand out in a pile of other résumés. You could have it printed in fancy type on shocking pink paper with a color copy of your photo at the top — but does such a résumé convey the non-verbal message you want to send? Such a résumé might be useful if you are applying to an ad agency or talent bureau, but most health care employers expect a more professional approach from nurses. For most health care employers, your résumé should be short, clear, well organized, and neat so that the essential points can be assessed quickly.

You need to consider some important things about yourself as a source. If you are looking for a job in a tight job market, you may need to send out several résumés at once. If your budget is slim, you may wish to develop one general résumé that can be photocopied and used for several potential employers, such as several hospitals in an urban area. If you use a computer, you may wish to develop a good general format, but adapt each résumé to fit the needs of each potential employer, such as a pediatric ward, a home care agency, or a geriatric facility.

If you do not deliver your résumé in person or attach it to a job application, you should attach a *covering letter*. The main message of this brief business letter simply says, using the appropriate words, that you are enclosing a résumé for consideration; if you are applying for a specific job, you can add information such as "I would like to apply for the position in your operating room that was recently advertised in *Canadian Nurse*." However, the covering letter also allows you to send the résumé to a particular person (and, as we said under the comments on business letters, it is always a good idea to write to a person rather than just a department or a general agency address).

The covering letter also allows you to provide a bit of additional personal information and to indicate that you would like to have a job interview. You can add such information as the best times to telephone you or how to leave a voice mail so that you can return the call. This kind of information is not suitable in the résumé itself.

A résumé alone will not get you a job. The purpose of a résumé is to get you a job interview. Potential employers develop a short list of possible employees based on their résumés (or application forms), so you should know how to develop a good one and supply all the important information in one or two pages.

CONTENT FOR A RÉSUMÉ

Most résumés fall into one of two broad categories: chronological and functional. The chronological résumé is the most common and concentrates on supplying details about your educational and employment history. The functional résumé allows you to tell more about the various jobs you have held. You need to keep information suitable for both types in your résumé file because this material will be useful when you fill out applications for nursing positions and when you go to interviews. However, the basic content is similar for both and includes the following categories. Sample résumés are shown in Boxes 6.6 and 6.7.

Name, address, and telephone number

They should be given clearly at the top of the first page. You do not usually supply other personal information (e.g., marital status, family, age, weight, height, and so on) in the résumé, and never at the top.

Education

List the highlights of your education in chronological order, starting with the most recent educational preparation and working back. When you graduate and are applying for your first positions, you may want to include your high school graduation, although employers will generally assume that, if you have graduated from a college or university, then you have completed high school. As you determine whether to include high school graduation, think SMART: source (are you young, inexperienced, and applying for a first position, or are you older, experienced, and applying for a senior position?); message (is your educational experience or your work experience more important to this potential employer?); audience (would this information be relevant to this reader?); route (have you room to include all the details?); and tone (is this a full-length, formal application in which you should include all relevant information?).

BOX 6.6   Sample Chronological Résumé (New Graduate)

NOEL KANE, R.N.
Apt. 12 — 1812 Bayview Street
Surrey, B.C. V4B 0X0
Telephone: (604) 555-3238

Job Objective: Registered Nurse Staff Position, Surrey
District Hospital

Education:

2002   Registered Nurse Degree
School of Nursing
Chinook Community College
Sardis, B.C.

1999   High School Graduation (with honors)
Duke of Connaught Senior Secondary
South Surrey, B.C.

Work Background:

2001   (Feb.) — 2002 (June) Kitchen Assistant
(weekend relief) Sardis Memorial Hospital,
Sardis, B.C.

1999   (June–July) Kitchen Assistant
Sardis Memorial Hospital, Sardis, B.C.

Awards:

1999   University Women's Club (South Fraser
Branch) Ethel Singh Scholarship ($1,000
for further study)

Professional Memberships:

2001   Registered Nurses Association of B.C.
1996–2001 Canadian Student Nurses Association
(national vice-president, 2000-01)

References:
Mr. J. R. Toews R.R.3, Box 17, Sardis, B.C. V6M 0X1
(604) 555-2198

Mrs. Cheryl Jones   School of Nursing, Chinook Community
College, Sardis, B.C. V7K 1X0
(604) 555-2176, local 546

(Prepared August 2002)

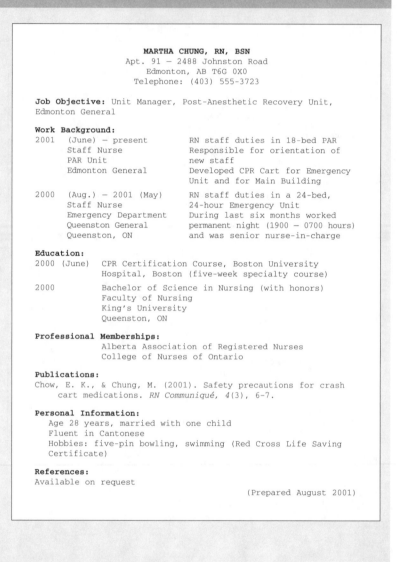

BOX 6.7   **Sample Functional Résumé (Recent Graduate)**

MARTHA CHUNG, RN, BSN
Apt. 91 — 2488 Johnston Road
Edmonton, AB T6G 0X0
Telephone: (403) 555-3723

Job Objective: Unit Manager, Post-Anesthetic Recovery Unit, Edmonton General

Work Background:

2001	(June) — present	RN staff duties in 18-bed PAR
	Staff Nurse	Responsible for orientation of
	PAR Unit	new staff
	Edmonton General	Developed CPR Cart for Emergency
		Unit and for Main Building
2000	(Aug.) — 2001 (May)	RN staff duties in a 24-bed,
	Staff Nurse	24-hour Emergency Unit
	Emergency Department	During last six months worked
	Queenston General	permanent night (1900 — 0700 hours)
	Queenston, ON	and was senior nurse-in-charge

Education:
2000 (June)   CPR Certification Course, Boston University
                    Hospital, Boston (five-week specialty course)

2000   Bachelor of Science in Nursing (with honors)
                    Faculty of Nursing
                    King's University
                    Queenston, ON

Professional Memberships:
                    Alberta Association of Registered Nurses
                    College of Nurses of Ontario

Publications:
Chow, E. K., & Chung, M. (2001). Safety precautions for crash
    cart medications. *RN Communiqué, 4*(3), 6-7.

Personal Information:
    Age 28 years, married with one child
    Fluent in Cantonese
    Hobbies: five-pin bowling, swimming (Red Cross Life Saving
    Certificate)

References:
Available on request

                                    (Prepared August 2001)

Information about relevant non-credit education may also be included in this section, such as information about short courses (e.g., CPR courses, or courses in operating room or neonatal care). You would definitely include information on certificate courses.

Work Experience

This section of your résumé will change most throughout your career. At first, you will not have much to include here, but you should regularly update your résumé files even if you do not need to develop a new résumé for each job.

If you are at an early stage in your career, you may wish to include information on part-time work even if it does not seem relevant to the job for which you are applying. One personnel officer told us that when he is reviewing for junior positions, he notes whether the applicant has worked summers at fast-food outlets such as McDonald's or A&W; he said that applicants who have managed to hold those jobs probably have a good overall work ethic. Sometimes volunteer work should be mentioned in this section as well; for example, if you worked every Thursday after classes throughout high school as a candystriper volunteer feeding patients in a geriatric ward of the hospital to which you are applying, you should include this information.

When you are further along in your career, you would list your various positions in chronological order, working back from the most recent. You could separate positions to mark advancements even though these positions were for the same employer. For example,

| 1996 — present | Unit Manager, Surgical Ward, Peace Arch Hospital, White Rock |
| 1994 — 1996 (Aug.) | Staff Nurse, Surgical Ward, Peace Arch Hospital, White Rock |

Later in your career, when you need to list several positions, you might combine these two.

Honors

In this section, which should be brief and to the point, you can include scholarships and awards.

Professional Memberships

You need to include information on your nursing registration and to indicate in which province(s) you are registered. If you are hired, you will need to provide your registration number, but as this is an important and confidential number we suggest that you do not put it on the résumé. Because provincial registration implies membership in the Canadian Nurses Association, you can decide whether to mention this membership or not. You should include all current professional memberships, and you may elect to include some or all past professional memberships. For example, if you held office in a professional nursing association in another province but are no longer a member, this information may still be relevant because it indicates involvement in professional activities. You would not usually include membership in civic, church, or social groups unless you believe that they are relevant to your audience and your message.

Publications

In this section, you list all your professional publications. Early in your career, you may not have many. If you eventually go into nursing education, the list of publications will likely be much longer. You must not trim this section in later years; a list of publications should be complete and uncensored — even if an article eventually seems immature or unimportant. In later years, you may wish to put a lengthy publication list on separate sheets and attach them only when relevant.

Personal Information

This section creates controversy. You are not required to give information such as age, marital status, or number of children, but sometimes this information is relevant (see example of the functional résumé). For example, if you are seeking a daytime job because you have a child and wish to be home in the evenings, you may want to make this point on your résumé (and in your covering letter). Many people believe that information about hobbies should never be included on a résumé — and that is appropriate for them as sources! Sometimes, however, information about extracurricular activities gives a potential employer an idea of the person behind the facts. Obviously, you have to think SMART and make up your own mind.

References

The inclusion of references with a résumé is another controversial point. Some agencies require that you supply them; others prefer to get in touch with one or more of your previous employers directly. It is certainly appropriate to say "References available on request," or you can simply omit this section. If you do use names, you should first ask the individuals if they are willing to give you a good recommendation.

Date

All résumés should be dated at the bottom of the page to ensure that an old one is not considered current. You need not sign the résumé.

POINTS TO REMEMBER ABOUT RÉSUMÉS

- Be accurate and truthful. Some prospective employers check the information. Furthermore, your résumé may form part of your permanent work record. Do not exaggerate responsibilities or try to oversell yourself!
- Be as brief as possible. One page is good; two full pages are maximum (even for senior administrators). Applicants for teaching positions at universities may use longer résumés.
- Double-check grammar, spelling, and punctuation. Use action words (e.g., developed, co-ordinated, supervised) when possible. Use point form or short paragraphs and the same verb tense throughout.
- Pay attention to visual presentation. A résumé should never look cramped — and should never be soiled or messy.
- Use a covering letter.
- Never underestimate yourself. A résumé is an advertisement for you; it is intended to get you an interview.

REPORTS

Reports are another standard way to send a message. They require the same SMART thinking and follow the same PROCESS as other written communications. The message, of course, could be delivered in many formats, but the report route is used when the message is longer and requires more detailed background than in a memo or letter. The tone tends to be more formal, although a report can range from slightly informal (between two colleagues working on a project) to highly formal (a royal commission report to a federal or provincial government). The audience can vary from a single individual to the general public, although reports tend to be shared with larger groups, so there is a primary audience (the person or small group who requested the report) and a secondary audience (the larger group with whom the primary audience may share the report). For a royal commission report, the person to whom the report is addressed in the covering letter may be the prime minister, but if the report is approved and released by the government, it may appear as a publication for the Canadian public. An annual report from a unit manager to the vice-president of nursing may end up being shared with the executive committee, the financial department, and the president of the hospital auxiliary, and may even be reproduced in the hospital's annual report to the public. Hence, a good starting point for a person asked to prepare a report is to find out exactly who needs the report and what its purpose is to be.

In other words, if you are asked to prepare a report, you need to follow the writing PROCESS — especially the first three steps at the bottom of the ladder. As part of your research, get copies of previous reports that may help you to understand the particular format used for that kind of report in your agency, but get other kinds of reports as well so that you can make innovative and creative changes. Obviously, if you are a hospital unit manager preparing a quarterly report, you will keep it simpler in format and layout than if you are an advertising agency manager preparing an annual report for the shareholders of Canada's largest bank.

Remember, however, that the message continues to be the point of a written communication. Be certain that you understand the message and its purpose. Are you asked to provide a report with data on various brands of infant cots so that a committee of several head nurses can make a decision? Or are you asked to recommend the brand of infant cots that should be purchased based on *your* research and expertise? In the former, you will need to provide all the background details on the various infant cots available, including costs, safety factors, ease of use, and other such details, so that the committee can debate the issue and make an informed decision; the purpose of the research report is to save the committee time. In the latter, you can be much more direct and brief and state that, based on your research and testing and after consideration of prices, you (an expert source) recommend the "Babe Cot" as the most suitable of six cots currently on the market. You might choose to support your recommendation briefly in the report and to include appendices that give background information on all the cots, but the main body of the report should be brief, to the point, and based on your expertise, because the purpose of your report is to *recommend*. In the latter instance, the committee might simply approve your report and send it on to the purchasing department — so you should include all the details the matériels manager will need to go ahead and make the order.

For reports in which you are asked to give an opinion or recommendation, you can use the acronym PRESS:

Position: state your position clearly.
Reason: state the reason you are for or against.
Example: give an example or two to illustrate your position.
Support: support your position with statistics and facts.
Summarize: close with a brief summary of your position.

Some reports fall halfway between the informational report and the recommendation report; these are termed "interpretive reports," which not only inform and describe but also analyze. The interpretive report, however, does not usually make recommendations. Progress reports fall into this category.

Proposals, including grant proposals and project requests, also come under the category of reports. Important sections of these reports include proposed costs (budget) and methods of implementation; a time schedule is also useful. If you are applying for a grant from a foundation, each one usually has specific forms that are used; check with the foundation before starting work (i.e., during the planning step of the PROCESS ladder). As part of planning, you may also want to borrow (or, if report writing is going to be a major part of your job, even buy) a book on how to write reports. Yes, there are books on how to write reports and even on how to write certain kinds of reports (e.g., writing proposals or writing technical reports). This section provides only an overview of reports. You should also review Appendix B to find recommended books on reports.

FORMAT OF A REPORT

A good report follows the traditional outline described in detail earlier in this book. The essentials are introduction, body, and conclusion. There is one slight difference, however. In most written communications, the introduction merely "Tells them what you are going to tell them" — and it does so in broad terms. In a report, the introduction *summarizes* what you are going to tell your audience and is specific about conclusions, recommendations, and actions to be taken. In other words, you give the essence of the report on the first page.

You provide a summary at the beginning because of the audience. For many readers of a business report, the summary is all that is required. If the reader needs more details, he or she can go deeper into the report — but most readers do not want to read the whole report to discover "the bottom line." Furthermore, the organization of the body of the report is based on this premise: you make it easy, through the organization, for a reader to find the details he or she needs.

If you hand out reports during a meeting, and the chair allows the members time to look at the report, observe how they react. Typically, about 80% of committee members will turn quickly to page 1 and start to read. If the opening on page 1 catches their interest with some solid information, they will continue to read all of page 1 and turn to page 2. About 40% of typical committee members continue to read page 2 (provided that the message stays relevant); the other 60% let their attention wander and may even start flipping through the rest of the report (many will turn to the end to look for conclusions there) or turn to other committee matters. Only about 10% will continue to read on to page 3. The same pattern is followed when people get your report in their offices; about 80% of them turn immediately to page 1. Depending on their time and the importance of the report to them, they will stay with it for page 2 and maybe page 3 — and then set the report aside to read when they have more time (which, for most busy people, is never). Thus, where should you put the important message in your report?

In the 1970s, reports typically started with all the background, went through the history of why the report was needed, and built up to the conclusion on the last few pages. Today, reports start with conclusions and recommendations, followed by the reasons for the recommendations, and the background and historical perspective (if included at all) tend to be near the end. The former style is still used occasionally, usually for expository or traditional reports; the latter style is considered motivational and is more likely to be used in hospitals and health care agencies.

The standard organization for a detailed report would thus follow this route (you will probably notice similarities to the student assignments described earlier in this book):

- **cover** (if necessary), with a good, catchy title;
- **title page(s)**, including information on authors or compilers, place, date, and other relevant material;
- **preliminary pages**, including table of contents (and perhaps a list of tables, graphs, or illustrations if used) if the report is more than 20 pages; in major reports, you may also need a preface and acknowledgments (but keep them brief);
- **introduction** — frequently entitled "Executive Summary" — in which the report is summarized in one or at most two pages; the introduction may even be put before the preliminary pages to make it stand out;
- **body of report**, which includes some or all of these elements:
  - synopsis or abstract of the body;
  - background (the why of this report);
  - method used to look into the subject (how you did it);
  - findings (with *all* the facts, including financial information);

- discussion (including your interpretation of the facts, your recommendations in detail, and your conclusions in detail);
- concluding section of the body (which ties the whole report together and reiterates the executive summary);
- **references and bibliography**; and
- **appendices** (*after* references and bibliography because usually they are attachments that you did not write).

Not all reports will follow this format, of course; it depends on Source * Message * Audience * Route * Tone. For example, some hospital administrations require quarterly and annual reports from department heads and have strict rules about format. One hospital vice-president asked her department heads to organize their quarterly reports this way:

1. Brief introductory statement followed by sections on progress since the last report (were goals met?)
2. Body giving statements and comparison figures on
   2.1 budget
   2.2 staffing
   2.3 administrative problems
   2.4 in-service education activities
   2.5 committee participation
   2.6 other relevant activities
3. Concluding section that includes a list of new long-term and short-term goals.

This vice-president also wanted her department heads to use a modified Harvard numbering style whereby each section in the body of the report used her specific numbering system and each paragraph in each section had a number. Thus, the first paragraph in the budget section was 2.1.1, the second paragraph was numbered 2.1.2, and so on. The department heads knew exactly what was expected by this particular audience and could prepare their reports accordingly.

SHORT REPORTS ("BRIEFS")

The term "brief" came into business use during the 1990s. Generally speaking, a brief is a *short* report usually recommending some kind of action or some solution to a problem. The term has been around much longer in the legal profession, in which a brief is a concise statement intended to inform other, usually more senior, counsellors about a client's case. No doubt you have also heard the term used in military circles in the form "briefing." The idea is to get a summary of a lot of information into a short, usable form for someone who knows less about a subject than you do but who is in a position to take action.

Professional associations often present briefs to political committees or commissions. A written brief or short report is taken to the committee's meeting, and a representative of the association gives an even briefer oral presentation and answers questions (e.g., to a royal commission on health care and costs). In these instances, a brief is a longer and more formal document than a letter or memo; a brief might contain 750 to 1,000 words (three to five pages), which would be a l-o-n-g letter!

The shortest reports can be sent as memos. For example, if a senior nurse administrator in your hospital asks you for a report on the status of a grant given to your department by the hospital auxiliary, he or she probably does not want a formal layout. An example of a short progress report sent as a memo is given in Box 6.8.

AGENDAS AND MINUTES

At some point in your career, you are likely going to be asked to "do" the minutes of a meeting — and good luck, especially if you are asked to do this at the last moment without any warning! Minutes are, in essence, one kind of report; they report on what happened during a meeting, and they generally reflect the action taken by the group (what was *done* rather than what was said). Names of movers of motions are generally required, and it may also be the style of the group to include the names of seconders. Some groups record only whether a motion passed or failed; others wish to have the numbers of people who voted for or against, or who abstained; still other groups record the names of those who voted for or against, or who abstained. The tone will vary from highly formal to informal, depending on the group, but generally should sound professional and businesslike.

Unfortunately, the rules of the route for minutes are almost as varied as meetings themselves. Minutes vary from full transcripts, such as Parliament's *Hansard*, of everything that was said in a meeting (long and complex, and they should only be assigned to a trained secretary who can take shorthand) to the sketchiest of communiqués that give only the motions (with movers and seconders) and a simple statement of whether the motion passed or failed. Other minutes provide a summary of the discussion that occurred on each motion and a summary of the committee reports. Still other types of minutes include complete copies of all reports by officers, committee chairs, and other speakers (supplied by these individuals).

BOX 6.8   Sample Short Progress Report (Memo Format)

 Well Known Hospital
54321 Major Drive
Well Known City, BC V4Z X0O
Telephone (604) 555-1234

TO: Jane Doe, Vice-President Patient Services
FROM: John Singh, RN, Unit Manager OR   **PHONE:** local 123
DATE: 16 March 2002

RE: Progress Report on WKH Auxiliary Special Funding

The Operating Room received a one-time special grant of $13,000 from the WKH Auxiliary in December 2001 to purchase operating room instruments. The purchase is progressing on time and on budget, with instruments worth $11,769 (including relevant taxes, delivery, and so on) ordered and received. When one more back order is received, the rest of the money will have been used.

Background

At a meeting of WKH OR staff, a list was drawn up of instruments often requested by surgeons but unavailable or in short supply. These instruments were in addition to those requested in the 2000–2001 OR budget; some items that had to be cut from the budget were included in this list.

OR staff then prepared a proposal for funding, in consultation with the Materiels Manager. The proposal was supported by the WKH Medical Committee and approved by WKH Administration. The funding proposal was submitted to the WKH Auxiliary in November, and the Auxiliary approved the $13,000 request at its meeting in early December.

The list included
- instruments for specialty work in ear surgery now that this specialty surgery is available at WKH;
- additional basic instruments to help shorten turn-around times for operations.

Orders to Date

On 13 January 2002, three magnifying lenses and a complete set of auricular instruments, including pinna scrapers, antihelix retractors, ossicle retrievers, and tympani forceps, were ordered from Ear-Ache Instruments of Toronto. These instruments arrived 12 February 2002. One of the magnifying lenses was

BOX 6.8   **Sample Short Progress Report (continued)**

scratched on arrival and has been returned; a replacement is on
its way. All other instruments were checked and incorporated
into OR stocks. Total cost of these instruments was $10,343.

A list of 12 special retractors often requested by surgeons
was drawn up by OR staff and checked with the Chief of Surgery.
The order was placed 19 January 2002 with Retractor-Magic of
Montreal and received 19 February. Total cost was $1,426.

An OR micro-sterilizer for auricular instruments has been
ordered through 3X Instruments of Boston (there is no Canadian
supplier). The list price is $987 (US); this should use most of
the remaining funds but remain within the funding budget.
Expected date of delivery is 20 March 2002. Final cost will
depend on the exchange rate when the order is received. If the
cost exceeds the $13,000 grant, the few extra dollars will be
taken from the general OR budget for supplies.

Copies of the purchase orders for all items, with prices,
are attached for information.

Future Actions

All equipment should be received and in use by 5 April 2002.

Once all equipment is received and put into use, letters
from the OR Head Nurse, the Chief of Surgery, and the new ENT
Specialist will be written and sent to the WKH Auxiliary
President outlining the use and thanking members for the grant.

Copy: J. Hancock, Materiels Manager

JS/sac

Points to note

A memo format was used for this response to a request for a (written) progress report on the use of the Auxiliary's money. Although it is only two pages long, it still likely tells Jane Doe more than she needs to know. However, it provides all the information that she may need if she has to discuss the matter with the Auxiliary president — or for whatever other reason that she wanted a written progress report (and not just a quick reply over the telephone). It even includes some review material to help remind her of the background.

Although it uses a long (8.5" x 11") memo form (which tends to make it somewhat informal in tone), John Singh arranged to have it typed for him (note the typist's initials), which makes it more formal. Furthermore, the single-spaced typed version fits onto two pages; a handwritten version would likely require more pages. As well, the language and the writing style tend to be formal.

Our best advice in a situation where you are asked, without warning, to take minutes is to discuss the style briefly with the chair, then take as complete a set of notes as possible. Later, obtain copies of minutes of several previous meetings of that group and follow the format and style used in those.

On the other hand, if you are going to be the designated recorder for a series of meetings, then we suggest you obtain guidelines from the organization involved. If such guidelines are not available, do some research in the library or on the Internet and, in conjunction with the person appointed to chair the meetings, work out the style of minutes that you believe would best suit this particular group. In other words, think SMART. It is truly important to work with the chair for the meeting, because an agenda (outline, usually numbered in point form, of the things to be discussed) is enormously helpful to the person who takes the minutes; the minutes will then follow the same headings as the agenda. The agenda usually is prepared by the chair of the group, but for some groups it may be the responsibility of the secretary.

Robert's Rules of Order (see Zimmerman, 1997), the accepted standard for conduct of official meetings in Canada, identifies the following basic items for an agenda:

1. Call to order
2. Approval of Agenda
   2.1 Addition 1 (list as many as required)
   2.2 ...
3. Approval of Minutes of Last Meeting(s)
4. Business Arising from Minutes
   4.1 First item from minutes (list as many as required)
   4.2 ....
5. Officers' and Committee Reports (e.g., chair, treasurer, committee heads)
   5.1 First report (list as many as expected to report)
   5.2 ...
6. Unfinished Business (e.g., items tabled or referred from previous meetings)
   6.1 First item (list as many as needed)
   6.2 ...
7. New Business (should have been identified to the chair before meeting, or added to agenda at opening)
   7.1 First new item (list as many items as needed)
   7.2 ...
8. Approval of Date of Next Meeting
9. Adjournment

The minutes would generally follow the same format, but *Robert's Rules* identifies several points that must be covered:

- Name of the group (or committee or section of the group)
- Kind of meeting (e.g., regular, special, board, committee)
- Date and place of meeting, and time meeting opened
- Presence of the regular presiding officer (chair) and secretary or, in either's absence, of the substitute
- Indication of who attended the meeting (which may simply be a statement that there was a quorum present, or the total number attending, or a full list of names of those attending and those who did not attend)
- Approval (with corrections, if any) of minutes of previous meeting — or, in some circumstances, their postponement until later (this latter may require a motion)
- All main motions, amendments, points of order, and appeals and whether these passed or failed or were withdrawn
- Reports given by committee chairs (with names) or other individuals and any actions taken
- Special announcements (e.g., related meetings, relevant actions by other groups)
- Time of adjournment.

The format for the minutes again varies, depending on the group's wishes and the style designed by the secretary. The notes may be in point form, or (more rarely) written in narrative paragraphs. Some groups call for minutes to be prepared in columns showing: Item of business, Person designated as responsible, and Action required. Other groups have three columns: Item, Points of discussion, and Action (including the name of the person responsible for taking the action and reporting back). If you are the secretary of a group, such as the nursing students' association, you may want to consider setting up a template or standardized format in a laptop computer that you can take to the meeting.

All minutes should be properly typed, signed, and preserved in a binder or other suitable form so they may be kept for future reference by the group, its members, and appropriate others.

HELPFUL HINTS ABOUT REPORTS

- Keep your report as short as possible — the briefer the better.
- Summarize your message on page 1.
- Keep the body of your report as brief as possible; use tables to summarize and present information visually; put background details into appendices.

- Keep the purpose of the report in mind — is it to inform, persuade, request, analyze, or recommend?
- Do you want the receivers of the report to take action? If so, be specific about the action you want them to take, and request it on page 1.
- Recommend solutions if you identify problems.
- Provide full information related to cost if relevant; in today's world, report readers are concerned about budgets.

RESEARCH PAPERS AND THESES

If you are in the final years of a baccalaureate nursing degree program or in a program for your master's degree, you may be asked to prepare a research paper, which represents another specialized route with many rules. The fifth edition of the *Publication Manual of the American Psychological Association* (APA, 2001) provides an overview. Two other excellent resources are *How to Write and Publish a Scientific Paper* (fourth edition), by Robert A. Day (1993), and *How to Teach Scientific Communication*, by F. Peter Woodford, published for the Council of Science Editors (1999). Other resources are identified in Appendix B.

As a route, a research paper (sometimes called a research report) follows many of the rules already described in this book for student assignments and reports. Sometimes a thesis is actually a research report. To prepare a research report, as with all written communications, you need to implement the SMART essentials and follow the writing PROCESS.

A research paper reports on the findings of a research project; usually, the writer is the principal researcher or a member of the research team that planned and carried out the project. By the time you are asked to prepare a research paper, you will have read numerous research reports and articles, and you will have taken or will be taking a course on the development of a research project.

Most likely, the project itself will start with the development of a research question or problem. Students often agonize over the evolution of a good research question. An excellent place to find one is in a nursing setting; ask staff nurses what problems they find in their day-to-day work, and then pose those problems as a research question. The preparation of the research question itself is a major task; if you do a good job of it, you will find it much easier later to write the research article or report.

It is crucial that you do research on the question itself before you commit yourself to a project. Eventually, you will write an abstract summarizing the research question and get it approved before you begin the project. You may also need to write a funding proposal related to the research project. Once you start looking into background material for the project, you will write up a literature review. Once you have done the review, you will need to identify the method that you are going to use in the written communication. Every step of the research process involves a new written communication. You may actually write up many of the stages as you proceed through the project. Once you have carried out the research, you are ready to prepare the final report.

FORMAT OF A RESEARCH PAPER

Most research reports follow the traditional, rigid scientific method of organization, which has become known as IMRAD, an acronym for Introduction, Method, Results, And Discussion. It follows the same format, with a few variations, as that already described for reports and student assignments. Many of the variations depend on the audience — the instructor for your course or the supervisor of your thesis committee. However, in general, the following show a basic format for a research paper, although the order of items will depend on the expectations of your audience:

- **title page** — usually has some rigid rules: it is longer and more formal in tone, and the title must accurately describe the contents of the paper so that it can be retrieved easily in a literature search; usually, there is no cover for a research paper, so the title page includes name(s) and title(s) of author(s) or project team, as well as address, date, and other relevant material;
- **preliminary pages**, including the table of contents, a list of tables, graphs, or illustrations, and perhaps a preface and acknowledgments;
- **abstract** — which is written last and which summarizes the project and report, although it may or may not give details of the findings (depending on the interpretation of your instructor); there may be a restriction on the length of the abstract (e.g., 125 words maximum, or one page maximum), and an abstract rarely takes more than two pages;
- **body of research paper**, which includes some or all of these elements:
  - introduction (which may be labelled as such in a research paper; includes history of or background to the project);
  - statement of research question/hypothesis/objectives of the study;
  - literature review;
  - research method(s) used (may include subsections on design, sample, data collection, and methods for analyzing data);
  - statement on human rights protection or other approvals needed;
  - statement on limitations of the study (may be positioned after results or as a subsection under the conclusion);

- results/findings (what you found out, with *all* the facts, including all statistical data);
- discussion/interpretation (your analysis of and comment on the facts in detail; may require subsections in a long study);
- conclusions (if the project reached any; they may be included under the discussion section);
- recommendations/applications (if the project reached any; they may be included under the discussion section or under the conclusion section);
- concluding section for the body of the research report (may be omitted if you let the conclusions and recommendations themselves end and round out the paper); and
- appendices (in a research paper or thesis, they come before the references and bibliography because usually you prepare any appendices);
- **references and bibliography**; and
- **index** (may be required, although this is a new idea).

HELPFUL HINTS FOR RESEARCH PAPERS/THESES

- If this is a student project, discuss **everything** with your instructor (or thesis committee) as early as possible in the project and regularly as you proceed.
- Preparation of these papers is usually a massive project, so break it down into small stages, with deadlines, and never leave it until the last minute.

ARTICLES

At some time in your nursing career, you may want to write an article for a professional journal; nurses often want to share good ideas with other nurses. The basic SMART elements and the writing PROCESS will also help you to prepare a good article that has a chance of being accepted by the editor and published in the journal.

As you contemplate the SMART elements, carefully consider yourself as a source. Can you speak authoritatively? Would someone be interested in your views on the subject? You can write an article as a student as long as you provide a student's viewpoint or interpretation. If you have spent a year or more researching a specific topic and gathering data that are new and pertinent, then you can write as a researcher. If you are elected as an officer of an association, you may be able to write on behalf of the members of that association. Just be sure that you recognize your role in writing the article.

The route will be a certain journal, so you need to be familiar with that journal. Look at its guidelines and format to see whether your message will be appropriate. Once you really look at professional journals as a possible author, you will discover that there are many different kinds (e.g., research journals, general interest journals, specialty journals, newsletters, abstract journals) and that within any one journal there are often different kinds of articles (e.g., news items, letters to the editor, editorials, opinion articles, general articles, research articles, book reviews). More than 100 professional journals are published specifically for nurses, and nearly 300 other professional journals in related fields accepted articles from nurses. Which journal and which type of article would be best suited to your message? To see the range of professional journals, visit the journals section of a large biomedical library. The library in your professional nurses' association headquarters usually carries a wide range of nursing journals, and the librarian there can provide you with a list of current nursing journals.

You also need to consider the readership of the journal, which will eventually make up your audience. If your message is directed to physicians, it will not be accepted if you send it to a nursing journal; for example, *Canadian Nurse* is not likely to accept an article telling doctors that they need to write more legibly. Some journals are directed to all registered nurses in a particular region (e.g., *Canadian Nurse*, or the journal published by a provincial nurses' association or union). Others have special audiences, such as nursing administrators (e.g., *Canadian Journal of Nursing Leadership*) or those interested in nursing research (e.g., *The Canadian Journal of Nursing Research / Revue canadienne de recherche en sciences infirmières*).

You can often gain a good understanding of the readers of the journal by reading the information, usually in small print, on the masthead. The masthead will also give you other information, such as the names of the editors, the address of the journal, its frequency of publication, its cost and whether it is sold by subscription or sent only to members, and, usually, whether it welcomes unsolicited manuscripts for review. Sometimes the masthead will tell you the number of copies that are printed for circulation and that you should write to the editors for guidelines and information before you submit an article.

As well, if you look through several issues of the journal, you will find that editors publish a page containing "Information for Authors" and sometimes a "Call for Papers" asking for articles related to specific topics. As a potential author, you should make careful note of these pages. (They may not be included in every issue, but they usually appear at least once a year.) The Information for Authors advises you about length and rules of the route and usually mentions which style guide should be followed.

You will also learn a great deal about the route and the audience simply by reviewing several copies of the journal for which you want to write. When you first begin to write articles for professional journals, it is a good idea to submit to a journal that you read regularly. If you review all the issues for the past year, you will get a good idea of recent topics and whether the tone is formal (as in most research journals) or slightly less formal (as in the journals for a general nursing audience, such as *Canadian Nurse* or *RN*). You could note whether the journal tends to use short, catchy titles or longer, research-oriented titles. You could see whether each article opens with an abstract. You could determine the messages that get published. You could notice the length of most articles (and even estimate the number of words on a page to give you an idea of length). You could check whether the journal uses photographs or not. All these points will affect how you eventually approach your message.

Most articles fall into one of these categories:

- research articles, which are similar to, but often shorter than, research reports;
- informational articles on procedures, processes, and techniques (often called "how to" articles);
- case studies, which describe in detail the care of a patient (either a typical or an unusual case); these reports used to be common in nursing journals but have been published less frequently in recent years;
- historical articles, which may or may not follow a special historical research format;
- articles on current issues, which are often called "opinion pieces" but which include some in-depth analysis of the various views on a new or controversial matter; and
- editorials, which are usually solicited by the staff of the journal.

We are not going to describe in detail the format and background for preparation of an article. There are a number of books (check Appendix B) and numerous articles on the Internet that deal with this topic. We are going to show you, however, a sample of a manuscript of a letter to the editor of a nursing journal written by a (fictional) student nurse with its attached covering letter (see Box 6.9). This example illustrates many of the points related to articles.

HELPFUL HINT FOR ARTICLES
- The briefer the better: short articles stand a much better chance of being accepted for publication than do long ones.

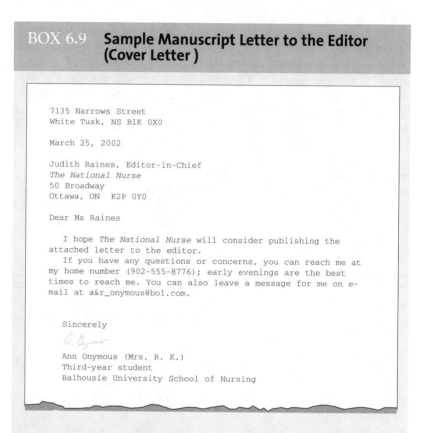

BOX 6.9   Sample Manuscript Letter to the Editor (Cover Letter)

7135 Narrows Street
White Tusk, NS B1K 0X0

March 25, 2002

Judith Raines, Editor-in-Chief
The National Nurse
50 Broadway
Ottawa, ON   K2P 0Y0

Dear Ms Raines

   I hope *The National Nurse* will consider publishing the
attached letter to the editor.
   If you have any questions or concerns, you can reach me at
my home number (902-555-8776); early evenings are the best
times to reach me. You can also leave a message for me on e-
mail at a&r_onymous@bol.com.

   Sincerely

   [signature]

   Ann Onymous (Mrs. R. K.)
   Third-year student
   Balhousie University School of Nursing

Points to note

Letters to the editor need to be formatted so that they can be handled
like a manuscript and sent for typesetting. As well, a published letter in
a professional journal usually does not contain a street address, only
the city; a covering letter giving address, phone number, and other
relevant details is therefore attached to the typescript for the letter to
be considered for publication.

BOX 6.9   Sample Manuscript Letter to the Editor (continued)

Networking Idea Letter to Editor — page 1

A Staff-and-Student Networking Idea

Opportunities for nursing students to network with practising registered nurses are vital but seem to be difficult to set up. However, RNs at Seal Cove District Hospital near Halifax, Nova Scotia, have involved students from the Balhousie Nursing Program in small, informal, practical network groups in a way that benefits both nurses and students.

For several years, staff nurses from the pediatric unit regularly met informally over coffee in the hospital cafeteria for one hour at the end of the day shift every other Thursday to exchange information on current nursing literature. Those who participated took turns reviewing current journals in the hospital's staff library and reporting to the group on articles of interest. Not all staff could attend every time, but several staff found the sessions valuable, and the meetings settled into a routine. The one-hour time limit was strictly observed.

About one year ago, these pediatric nurses invited students assigned to the ward to attend the meetings. The students proved enthusiastic participants, and some asked if they could continue to drop in after they finished the ward assignment. The staff nurses agreed, and the reading group has become larger, with three students interested in pursuing pediatric nursing becoming regular participants. These students have access through the university library to pediatric journals not regularly received in the hospital, and this access benefits the staff group. Students benefit from the regular friendly contact with practising nurses and from hearing practical discussions related to the literature.

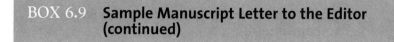

BOX 6.9   **Sample Manuscript Letter to the Editor (continued)**

Networking Idea Letter to Editor — page 2

Furthermore, the students have reported the idea in other departments, and two other "reading groups" have been set up at Seal Cove Hospital, one by nurses in the emergency department, and one by the geriatric staff; several students from Balhousie take part regularly. Nursing administration at the hospital has supported this informal continuing education project by supplying free coffee, tea, or juice for meetings of all three groups.

The Boundary Health Unit in Seal Cove also has set up a "Literary Lunch Bunch" and invites students assigned to the unit to take part. Unfortunately, few students can continue this involvement once the community health assignment is over, because the midday time conflicts with class schedules. At least one student, however, has been an off-and-on regular with this group for six months and now plans to follow a career in public health.

Nurses who participate in reading groups in other parts of Canada might want to consider including students. I know from experience that this form of networking is much appreciated.

Ann Onymous

Third-year student, Balhousie University

White Tusk, NS

More points to note

The typescript of a letter to the editor (or other possible item sent to a journal, such as a news item, book review, or classified ad) should be double spaced, with typical wide margins and each page clearly labelled with a running head and the page number. Follow the style guide required by the journal. You do not need to have a title page for a letter to the editor; the covering letter takes on this role for short items that probably will not be sent for peer review.

BOX 6.9   Sample Manuscript Letter to the Editor (continued)

Note the short paragraphs, which make reading easier. Letters in journals or newspapers are usually set in narrow columns, and even a short paragraph will look long in such a column.

Letters to the editor are one of the most popular sections in any journal and get the attention of a lot of readers. If you can keep your message relatively short (as in the 420-word letter above), it will likely attract more readers than will an article on the same subject.

The section for Letters to the Editor frequently has a word limit (often with a maximum word count of 450 words); check the beginning and end of the section in the journal to see if length is mentioned. Even if the journal does not specify length, keep the letter as short as possible; it is then more likely to be accepted for publication.

SUMMARY

Throughout your career as a nurse, you will need to prepare hundreds of written communications. Furthermore, the styles and formats of these written communications will likely change many times during your lifetime, largely because of changes in technology. For example, the layout of business letters has changed markedly during the last century; the first changes occurred when businesses switched from handwritten to typed letters. In the last 25 years, letter-writing styles have changed several times, largely because of the introduction of computers.

Because of computers, moreover, footnotes in essays could come back into fashion and replace the author–year style. In the future, more writers will submit their reports and articles electronically (e.g., on disk or by file transfer through e-mail). Computer software will likely improve so that margins are set and reset automatically. Already many nursing courses are offered over the Internet and all communication is electronic.

The format of reports will change because much information formerly compiled and kept by individual departments (e.g., staffing figures, patient census) will be available to qualified personnel through the agency's computer system. Submission of articles to journals will change as well. More and more online journals will appear, and they will likely accept manuscript submissions from authors through file transfer.

So, although the formats described in these chapters will be useful to you, the most important things to learn from the book are the application of the SMART elements of communication and the use of the writing PROCESS. Their principles will last for your lifetime. Once you have learned how to use these principles, you are on the road to growth as a writer, no matter how styles change.

A Guide to APA Style in Reference Lists and Bibliographies

This Guide explains the principles, purposes, and functions of the author–year reference style recommended in the *Publication Manual of the American Psychological Association*, fifth edition, published in 2001 by the American Psychological Association, Washington, DC. It provides examples of common forms of references that student nurses will use in their papers. It by no means replaces that 439-page resource, especially for students doing theses and dissertations or for nurses who wish to publish in journals requiring APA style. However, our Guide does provide additional background information (using real references to nursing or health materials) for those just starting to write college or university papers and for those not familiar with doing citations.

This appendix shows both how to include the author–year reference in the body of your paper and how to set up the reference in the reference list based on the complete citation you made when you were doing your research. (See Chapter 4 for information on what is included in a "complete citation.") Details vary considerably depending on the number of authors and on decisions about capitalization and punctuation style developed by APA editors over many years. There *is* a logic behind the ways that this is done and in the "points to notice" we will try to show you that logic so that you can eventually do many of your references without having to consult this Guide or the *Manual* every time. For more details and more complex examples, you should buy a copy of the *Manual*, consult it in your learning centre or library, or check Web sites that offer information about APA style.

Such sites include the American Psychological Association's own Web site at http://www.apa.org or one of the many other Internet sites that offer examples of APA style references (use a keyword search, such as "APA reference style").

Figure A.1 shows basic components for a reference for a (fictional) book and journal article written by only one author. Once you understand and become familiar with these basics, you should soon be able to do most citations readily and be able to combine elements from one example with another. For instance, the example showing how to list six or more authors for a journal article would also apply if there were six or more authors for a book, or for a chapter in a book, or for material retrieved online or in a limited-circulation document.

Documents obtained through the Internet share many of the same citation elements as print materials (e.g., authors, dates, titles) and are treated similarly to them. However, you must include the address and the date you retrieved the information. See Chapter 4 and Figure 4.1. for more about describing the address or path you used, including the complete *uniform resource locator* or URL. If you wish to mention a Web site, but not a specific document on the site, in the body of your paper, the site can be referred to in the body of the paper but need not be included in the reference list.

Finally, remember that personal communications, which include e-mail messages, are not included in the reference list. See Chapter 4 for more information about using personal communications and see the Sample Student Paper in Chapter 5 for examples on how to cite personal communications in the body of your paper.

Book, Single Author

```
Buckley, J. (1998). Fit to print: The Canadian student's
     guide to essay writing. (4th ed.). Toronto: Harcourt
     Brace Canada.
```

In body of paper: (Buckley, 1998); with a quotation: (Buckley, 1998, p. xx).

Points to notice: position of period in relation to parentheses; capitals are used only for first letters in each section of the title of a book and for proper nouns (note differences for journals below); the apostrophe in "student's" — be certain you have copied it correctly.

FIGURE A.1 **Components of an APA Style Reference**

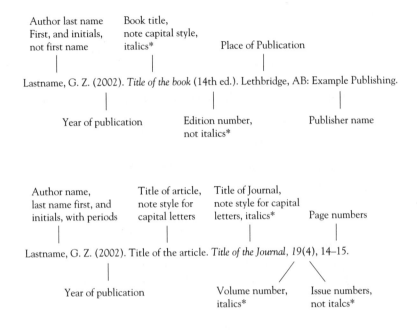

* You may use either underlining or the italic typeface on your computer. Underlining was a convention used in the days when manuscripts were prepared on typewriters to indicate that the material should appear in italics; now computers make it just as easy to show italic type as to show underlining.

Book, Two Authors

Zilm, G., & Warbinek, E. (1994). *Legacy: History of nursing education at the University of British Columbia 1919-1994.* Vancouver: University of British Columbia School of Nursing.

In body of paper: (Zilm & Warbinek, 1994); with a quotation: (Zilm & Warbinek, 1994, p. xx).

Points to notice: use of commas around authors' initials.

Book, Two Editors

Hibberd, J. M., & Kyle, M. E. (Eds.). (1994). *Nursing management in Canada*. Toronto: Saunders.

In body of paper: (Hibberd & Kyle, 1994); with a quotation: (Hibberd & Kyle, 1994, p. xx).

Point to notice: the period both inside and after the parentheses for "Eds."

Book, Two Editors, Second Edition

Hibberd, J. M., & Smith, D. L. (Eds.). (1999). *Nursing management in Canada* (2nd ed.). Toronto: Saunders Canada.

In body of paper: you probably would not refer to such material in the body of the paper because the chapters were written by different authors, and you need to give those authors' names; this would be a suitable listing in a bibliography; you might have to refer to this source in the unlikely event that you are using material from the preface.

Points to notice: compare this example with the one immediately above, which was the first edition, and you will note that one of the editors has changed; note capital *E* for "Eds." (editors), but small *e* for "ed." (edition).

Chapter in Edited Book, Three Authors

Field, P. A., Stinson, S. M., & Thibaudeau, M-F. (1992). Graduate nursing education in Canada. In A. J. Baumgart & J. Larsen (Eds.), *Canadian nursing faces the future* (2nd ed., pp. 421–445). Toronto: Mosby-Year Book.

In body of paper: (Field, Stinson, & Thibaudeau, 1992); with a quotation: (Field, Stinson, & Thibaudeau, 1992, pp. xx–xx).

Points to notice: commas around initials; the hyphen in Thibaudeau's initials, a convention for a hyphenated first name (Marie-France); position of initials for editors of the book; page numbers for the chapter given in parentheses after the book title and edition number; if there is a volume number, an edition number, and page numbers, these are all within one set of parentheses and separated by commas; use of abbreviation "pp." when page numbers for the chapter are given.

Book Reprinted From Original

Nightingale, F. (1946). *Notes on nursing: What it is, and what it is not.* Philadelphia: Lippincott. (Original work published 1859)

In body of paper: (Nightingale, 1946); with a quotation: (Nightingale, 1946, p. xx). But you should make it clear in the text that the original was published earlier through reference either to this well-known author or to the year the original appeared.

Point to notice: no period at the end of the citation.

Book, Group or Agency Author

American Psychological Association. (2001). *Publication manual of the American Psychological Association* (5th ed.). Washington, DC: Author.

In body of paper: if mentioned only once (American Psychological Association, 2001); with a quotation: (American Psychological Association, 2001, p. xx). If mentioned more than once, use (American Psychological Association [APA], 2001) for the first mention, then (APA, 2001) thereafter. When the group or agency is well known and frequently referred to by its initials (e.g., American Psychological Association [APA], Canadian Nurses Association [CNA], or World Health Organization [WHO]), and you are referring to it often in your paper, use the abbreviation.

Points to notice: postal code designations for provinces, states, and countries are not considered abbreviations and do not need periods; use of word "Author" when the publisher is the same agency that is the author of the material.

Book, Government Agency as Author

Statistics Canada. (1981). *Standard occupational classification 1980* (Catalogue 12-565E). Ottawa: Minister of Supply and Services Canada.

In body of paper: (Statistics Canada, 1981); with a quotation: (Statistics Canada, 1981, p. xx).

Point to notice: many government documents have either catalogue numbers or report numbers, and whenever possible they should be included (if your readers ever need to find the report, this number really helps a librarian track it down).

Book, No Publication Date Given

Brown, D. J. (n.d.). *The challenge of caring: A history of women and health care in British Columbia.* Victoria: British Columbia Ministry of Health and Ministry Responsible for Seniors, Women's Health Bureau.

In body of paper: (Brown, n.d.); with a quotation: (Brown, n.d., p. xx).

Points to notice: name of the government ministry that published the work has to be spelled out in full; n.d. — lower case letters and periods — stands for *no date.*

The preceding example is the way the APA (2001) *Manual* currently recommends. However, because a date of publication is important, especially in research, and because a date also is useful in finding material in library searches, many instructors prefer that you use a style that gives an approximate date. Thus, when you were doing your "complete citation" (see Chapter 4), you examine the book and try to estimate when it was published. As this book was purchased in 2000 and contains some 1999 data, the estimated date of publication is 2000. You would then do the listing this way:

Brown, D. J. (c2000). *The challenge of caring: A history of women and health care in British Columbia.* Victoria: British Columbia Ministry of Health and Ministry Responsible for Seniors, Women's Health Bureau.

In body of paper: (Brown, c2000); with a quotation: (Brown, c2000, p. xx).

Points to notice: the c before the year stands for *circa* (which means *about*) and is used when no date is given on the title or copyright page.

Book or Major Report, Government Ministry as Author

Manitoba Health. (1995). *The midwifery model of practice in Manitoba: Statement on midwifery*. Winnipeg: Government Printing Office.

In body of paper: (Manitoba Health, 1995); with a quotation: (Manitoba Health, 1995, p. x).

Points to notice: sometimes there might be periods to separate the names of the province or state, the ministry, and the department — as in the preceding example: British Columbia. Ministry of Health and Ministry Responsible for Seniors. Women's Health Bureau.; in this instance, the style within the body of the paper could be shortened to (British Columbia: Ministry of Health, c2000) unless there were several documents from the various departments of this ministry cited in your paper.

Journal Article, One Author, Paginated by Volume

Hawley, M. P. (1992). Sources of stress for emergency nurses in four urban Canadian emergency departments. *Journal of Emergency Nursing, 18*, 211–216.

In body of paper: (Hawley, 1992); with a quotation: (Hawley, 1992, p. xx).

Points to notice: capitals used for all major words in the title of a journal because it represents a proper name; underlining (or italics) for the title includes the volume number but not the page range.

Journal Article, One Author, Paginated by Issue

Wylie, D. M. (1996). Perspectives on the staff nurse [editorial]. *Canadian Journal of Nursing Administration, 9*(2), 5–6.

In body of paper: (Wylie, 1996); with a quotation: (Wylie, 1996, p. x).

Points to notice: information about a special kind of article (e.g., editorial, letter to the editor) is noted in brackets following the title; no spacing between volume and issue numbers.

Journal Article, Three to Five Authors

Cameron, S. J., Keil, J., Rajacich, D., & Dunham, K.
(1996). Using functional health patterns to predict
outcome with seniors. *The Canadian Nurse:
L'infirmière canadienne, 92*(10), 34-38.

In body of paper: on first mention (Cameron, Keil, Rajacich, & Dunham, 1996); with a quotation: (Cameron, Keil, Rajacich, & Dunham, 1996, p. xx). For subsequent mentions, use (Cameron et al., 1996) or (Cameron et al., 1996, p. xx), unless there is more than one article published in 1996 by a group of authors headed by Cameron. If this happens (albeit rarely in student papers), then you need to list as many authors as is necessary to distinguish between the two citations; this number may be two, followed by "et al.," or it may be the whole list.

Points to notice: use of period in "et al."; full name of journal used; note the lack of capitals in the French-language name, which is the way it is used as a proper name by this particular journal.

Journal Article, More Than Six Authors

Cilistka, D., Mitchell, A., Baumann, A., Sheppard, K.,
Van Berkel, C., Adam, V., et al. (1996). Changing
nursing practice — Trisectoral collaboration in
decision making. *Canadian Journal of Nursing
Administration, 9*(2), 60-73.

In body of paper: even on first mention (Cilistka et al., 1996); with a quotation: (Cilistka et al., 1996, p. xx), unless there are two or more citations for the same year with Cilistka as the first author. If there are (rare), then list as many authors as necessary, followed by "et al.," to distinguish between the two full citations.

Points to notice: in the reference list, you list the first six authors followed by "et al."; this article had eight authors (including Underwood, J., & Southwell, D.), and in a student paper you (source) could have decided to list them all in the reference list unless your instructor (audience) wished you to follow the style used for APA journals; within the body of the paper, you use the short form with "et al.," even on the first mention.

Journal Article, No Volume or Issue Number

Bauer, G. (2000, February). Your healthiest year ever. *Chatelaine*, pp. 50-52, 54, 57.

In body of paper: (Bauer, 2000); with a quotation: (Bauer, 2000, p. xx).

Points to notice: the month is not abbreviated; the abbreviation "pp." is used before page numbers; the comma in this page number sequence indicates that the pages are not continuous — that is, the article runs on pages 50 to 52, but something else (maybe an ad) is on page 53, and the article continues on page 54 and concludes on page 57.

Newsletter Article, No Author Named

Nursing remedies from head to toe. (2001, Spring). *History of Nursing News* [Newsletter of the BC History of Nursing Professional Practice Group], p. 9.

In body of paper: ("Nursing remedies ...," 2001); with a quotation: ("Nursing remedies ...," 2001, p. 9). If the title is short (two or three words), use the whole title, still with quotation marks; if the title is long, use the first two or three words followed by an ellipsis of three dots.

Points to notice: when no author's name is given with an article, it is harder to use the author–year style; when this happens, the first element of the reference is the title; within your paper, you also identify the article by a shortened version of its title, followed by the year; the complete title is given in the reference list.

Videotape or Film

British Columbia Nurses' Union. (c1992). *As hearts turn* (Video). (Available from B.C. Nurses' Union, 100 – 4259 Canada Way, Burnaby, BC V5G 1H1).

In body of paper: (B.C. Nurses' Union, c1992); it is unlikely that you would use a direct quotation from the film, but if you do, you do not need to specify a point on the film; if more than one reference to this video in the paper, use (B.C. Nurses' Union [BCNU], c1992) on first mention and (BCNU, c1992) for subsequent mentions.

Points to notice: abbreviation of British Columbia to B.C., which is suitable if you are writing within Canada for a Canadian audience, but it needs to be spelled out if you are writing for an American journal; use of periods when B.C. is an abbreviation, but not in the postal code designation; use of the apostrophe, which is part of BCNU's proper name; use of c1992, because there is no date given on this tape; use of the full address, although it may not be necessary for some audiences, in which case you would just say (Available from B.C. Nurses' Union).

Unpublished or Limited-Circulation Documents

Zilm, G. (1994). *The write way: A distance education work book*. Unpublished course material, University of Victoria School of Nursing Distance Education in Nursing Program, Victoria, BC.

In body of paper: (Zilm, 1994); with a quotation: (Zilm, 1994, p. xx).

Points to notice: similar to other unpublished documents such as theses; the city comes after the place where the unpublished material was presented, distributed, or stored.

Unpublished Course Syllabus or Printed Course Materials

Bramadat, I. (1995, January). *49:703 Course syllabus: Foundations, issues & trends in nursing*. Unpublished course syllabus, University of Manitoba School of Nursing, Winnipeg, MB.

In body of paper: (Bramadat, 1995); in the rare instance that you use a direct quotation from such material: (Bramadat, 1995, p. x). Note that if you are quoting or paraphrasing from a lecture itself (no printed notes), you treat this as a *personal communication* (see Chapter 4), which is fully described in the body of the paper and is not listed in the reference list.

Points to notice: the punctuation, including the ampersand (&), in the title is copied exactly from the title used in the course syllabus; do not necessarily follow the style you use in your own documents.

Material From a CD-ROM

Tynes, L. L. (1993). Tuberculosis: The continuing story. *JAMA: Journal of the American Medical Association, 270*, 2616-2617. Retrieved from InfoTrac Database Health Reference Center, CD-ROM, July 1992–July 1995 (available Guildford Public Library, Surrey, BC)

In body of paper: (Tynes, 1993); even if you use a direct quotation, you cannot usually give a page number because the file printed out on your printer will be in a different format; it is possible to use (Tynes, 1993, ¶xx).

Points to notice: this example is taken from a CD-ROM from a company called the Health Reference Center. It supplies disks monthly to subscribers (e.g., libraries, hospitals, wealthy individuals). Each new disk contains abstracts and sometimes complete texts purchased by this service from more than 300 professional medical and nursing journals and kept on the disk for the most recent three-year period. Readers can browse electronically through all these recent journals using keywords to find relevant articles and may then print out the abstract or, if available, the full text. For the article in this example, you might also obtain the original journal if it is available locally, although in the future much of this kind of material may be published only on CD-ROM or online. On some CD-ROMs (although not this one), each item has a file retrieval number; if so, it is given at the end of the item.

Article From Online Journal

Schloman, B. F. (2001, April). Nursing faculty and scholarly publishing: Survey of perceptions and journal use. *Online Journal of Issues in Nursing, 5*(1), manuscript 8. Retrieved May 25, 2001 from http://www.nursingworld.org/ojin/topic11/tpc11_8.htm

In body of paper: (Schloman, 2001); with a quotation: (Schloman, 2001, para. xx).

Points to notice: a reputable online journal (e-zine), although not all journals found in a keyword search might be reliable; note that this ending is "htm" (rather than "html" as in some citations) — be sure you copy correctly; no punctuation is used at the end of the specified path.

Document From Internet Site

American Psychological Association. (2001, January 10).
    Electronic reference formats recommended by the
    American Psychological Association. Washington, DC:
    Author. Retrieved May 24, 2001, from
    http://www.apa.org/journals/webref.html

In body of paper: (American Psychological Association [APA],
2001) on first mention, and (APA, 2001) on subsequent mentions; for a
quotation: (American Psychological Association, 2001, ¶ xx);
you may use page numbers rather than paragraph symbols if these are available — for example, (APA, 2001, p. 2 of 5); if you cannot use the
paragraph symbol (¶) you substitute the abbreviation "para." including the
period.

Points to notice: this citation is similar to that for a print document, but
the month and day in addition to the year in parentheses show when the site
was last updated and this should be given because Web sites are changed and
updated frequently; the date of retrieval (date you visited the site) is also
given, followed by the Web address (URL); you may break the URL address
following a slash.

Journal Abstract From Online Database

Krasner, D., & van Rijswijk, L. (1995). Research and
    writing basics: Elements of the abstract [Abstract].
    Ostomy/Wound Management, 41(3), 14, 16–17. Retrieved
    May 26, 2001 from http://www.rnabc.bc.ca/ using the
    CINHAL w/Heading database and keyword "abstracts"

In body of paper: treat similarly to a print journal item (Krasner & van
Rijswijk, 1995); with a quotation: (Krasner & van Rijswijk,
1995, online abstract l. x) with "l." standing for "line."

Points to notice: this example was taken from an online search accessed
through the Web site of the Registered Nurses Association of B.C.
(RNABC) where members can use a password to access a CINHAL database
(this one is called "with Headings") using the keyword "abstracts." We made
a printout (one page) of record 31 (of a possible 57 records); this page contained, among other useful data, a copy of the abstract (but not the article
itself), and the information that this journal (*Ostomy/Wound Management*)

was not available in the RNABC library. Other data available included information on the quality of the journal itself (e.g., expert peer reviewed). We could have tried to obtain the journal itself, but if it were not available locally, we might have wanted to paraphrase or quote some of the material from the online abstract (not always a good idea, but suitable in *some* student papers).

Information From a Private Organization Web Site

Canadian Federation of Nurses Unions. (2001). *Nurses salary chart, 2001: General duty registered nurses*. Retrieved August 27, 2001 from http://www.nursesunions.ca/ cb/index.shtml

In body of paper: (Canadian Federation of Nurses Unions [CFNU], 2001).

Points to notice: note "shtml."

Annotated Reference and Bibliography: Useful Readings/ Reference Tools

This *annotated* reference list and bibliography includes all chapter references, plus additional background books and articles. In it, we suggest useful reference tools for nurses who want to write more effectively. You can find many of the books mentioned in the Writing and References section of a college or university book store and in most college and university libraries. Some are "old" (such as the books by Theodore Bernstein), but are classics recommended and used frequently by professional writers. In some instances, you may find a later edition than the one mentioned here.

The style used in this list differs from the style recommended in the fifth edition of the *Publication Manual of the American Psychological Association* (American Psychological Association [APA], 2001); that style is illustrated in the Sample Student Paper on pages 115–124, in the annotated Working Bibliography on pages 96–97, and in the Reference examples in Appendix A on pages 175–187.

This annotated reference list differs in five main areas, all of which relate to SMART principles. First, this list gives full first names of authors as listed on their works because we (source) like to know and record first names; we included them to help make you (our audience) more familiar with some important expert writers and nursing leaders. The APA (2001) *Manual* recommends use of initials; full-name style takes more space, so editors of journals (the *Manual's* primary audience) do not like it. Second, the style also is changed because it is printed in a textbook (a different route than a typed student paper); APA recommends use of justified left-hand margins and ragged (not justified) right-hand margins. Textbooks are easier to read, and look much better, if both margins are justified. Because of this change in justification style, the experts who key manuscripts into type for a book will hyphenate words at the end of lines to avoid unsightly large spaces. Third, a sans serif font is used for each of these reference listings because this fits with the overall design of the book (route) and because it gives greater visual impact. Fourth, the indentation in the hanging indent is smaller than that recommended by APA, and the annotation is indented only once, because it saves considerable space (pages) in the book; APA style for papers and manuscripts calls for two indentations (the first of about five spaces and the second of about two spaces) as shown in the annotations in Box 4.1 on page 96–97. Fifth, because this *is* a book, the material is not double-spaced.

We hope that seeing these changes may help you understand more about SMART principles and about differences in finished copy in a typed student paper and a printed book.

American Psychological Association. (2001, January 10). *Electronic reference formats recommended by the American Psychological Association.* Washington, DC: Author. Retrieved May 24, 2001, from the World Wide Web: http://www.apa.org/journals/webref.html

One of the frequent computer updates related to changes and additions to the fourth edition of the APA *Manual.* This site regularly shows some of the latest ways of referencing electronic materials. Check this site and the APA home page — which is <www.apa.org/> regularly for updates and answers to questions about style.

American Psychological Association. (2001). *Publication manual of the American Psychological Association* (5th ed.). Washington, DC: Author.

The most useful style guide for nurses and nursing students. Buy a copy of the latest edition for your reference shelves as soon as you can afford one.

Avis, W. S., Drysdale, P. D., Gregg, R. J., Newfeldt, V. E., & Scargill, M. H. (1983). *Gage Canadian dictionary.* Toronto: Gage. (New printing 2000)

Excellent dictionary for Canadian students at the postsecondary level. In 2000–2001, this was reissued in an inexpensive softcover edition. A later edition (see de Wolf, Gregg, Harris, & Scargill, 1997, listed below) is available, but this first edition has an excellent introduction on reasons why a *Canadian* dictionary is important. You must have a good dictionary on your reference shelf even if you have a spell check-er in your computer.

Bernstein, Theodore M. (1971). *Miss Thistlebottom's hobgoblins: The careful writer's guide to the taboos, bugbears and out-moded rules of English usage.* New York: Farrar, Straus and Giroux.

A delightful book by a master writer; it reports on changes in English grammar, punctuation, and style. If you like writing and words and can find this — or *any* of Bernstein's books — in a library or second-hand store, savour it.

Bernstein, Theodore M. (1973). *The careful writer: A modern guide to English usage.* New York: Atheneum.

An old book, recently reprinted. A useful reference if you tend to misuse words. You may have to look for this in a second-hand bookstore, but it is a wonderful reference.

Buckley, Joanne. (1998). *Fit to print: The Canadian student's guide to essay writing* (4th ed.). Toronto: Harcourt Brace Canada.

An excellent reference tool with more detail on essay writing for arts courses, such as English, and with emphasis on errors of grammar and punctuation.

The Chicago manual of style for authors, editors, and copywriters (14th ed.). (1993). Chicago: University of Chicago Press.

A huge classic style manual that forms the basis for style for most book publishers; the first edition, published in 1906, was one of the first style guides. Many journals still recommend this style to their authors.

Colombo, J. R. (Ed.). (1974). *Colombo's Canadian quotations.* Edmonton: Hurtig.

This dictionary of quotations, alphabetically by author, includes 6,000 quotations all of which have some connection with Canada. It was just one of the useful reference tools that you may wish to add to your shelf some day.

Council of Biology Editors. (1994). *Scientific style and format: The CBE manual for authors, editors, and publishers* (6th ed.). New York: Cambridge University Press.

Another big style manual of the same genre as the APA *Manual*. Borrow it if you are writing for a journal that uses CBE style. Note that the Council of Biology Editors changed its name to the Council of Science Editors in 2000.

Cremmins, Edward T. (1982). *The art of abstracting.* Philadelphia: iSi Press, 1982.

A whole book on how to write an abstract! You can borrow it from a library when you come to work on the abstract for your master's thesis or for your doctoral dissertation. A 1993 edition is available but is expensive. Mentioned in Chapter 5.

Davies, Barbara, & Logan, Jo. (1999). *Reading research: A user-friendly guide for nurses and other health care professionals* (2nd ed.). Ottawa: Canadian Nurses Association.

An excellent, small, inexpensive pamphlet suitable for students just entering a nursing program. It helps you to know how to read, understand, and evaluate the quality of research articles published in professional journals.

Day, Robert A. (1993). *How to write and publish a scientific paper* (4th ed.). Phoenix, AZ: Oryx Press.

An excellent book to own if you really like to write and an essential if you are taking a master's degree or planning to publish an article.

Day, Robert A. (1995). *Scientific English: A guide for scientists and other professionals* (2nd ed.). Phoenix, AZ: Oryx Press.

An excellent reference tool for those in the final years of a university course or in graduate school. The first edition, 1992, might be available in second-hand stores and is just as useful.

de Wolf, G. D., Gregg, R. J., Harris, B. P., & Scargill, M. H. (1997). *Gage Canadian dictionary* (Rev. ed.). Toronto: Gage. (Later printings, marked 2000 on the cover, available)

The most recent edition (see above, Avis et al., 1983) of a good Canadian dictionary.

Donner, Gail J., & Wheeler, Mary M. (Eds.). (1998). *Taking control of your career and your future: For nurses, by nurses.* Ottawa: Canadian Nurses Association.

As well as some useful examples of résumés and some thoughtful comments on self-reflective journalling, this book contains useful background on changes in the workplace and will be useful for nurses throughout their careers.

Dupuis, K. Carew, & Wilson, S. V. (1982). *Communicating with P.O.W.E.R.* Toronto: Gage Publishing.

Old, and our text covers the same basic material, but Dupuis and Wilson give you another way to approach what we call the writing PROCESS. Mentioned in Chapter 2.

Elbow, Peter. (2000). *Everyone can write.* New York: Oxford University Press.

Elbow's first book, *Writing with power: Techniques for mastering the writing process* (1981), is also an excellent book if you are a good writer and want to be better. Both are available in most college and university bookstores and are recommended in many English departments.

Flesch, Rudolf. (1960). *How to write, speak, and think more effectively.* New York: New American Library.

Cited in Chapter 3. Flesch was one of the first communication gurus, and looked for scientific ways to measure "readability."

Furberg, Jon, & Hopkins, Richard. (2000). *College style sheet: Fifth Canadian edition.* Vancouver: 49th Avenue Press (Langara College).

This slim, inexpensive volume mentioned in Chapter 4 provides a summary of important points about style, including APA style, as well as brief explanations of most other style guides used at the college and university levels. It also provides excellent sample layouts for typing your papers.

Gordon, Karen Elizabeth. (1983). *The well-tempered sentence: A punctuation handbook for the innocent, the eager, and the doomed.* New York: Ticknor & Fields.

A fun-type reference with unique and memorable examples of punctuation errors, with advice on solutions.

Gordon, Karen Elizabeth. (1984). *The transitive vampire: A handbook of grammar for the innocent, the eager, and the doomed.* New York: Times Books.

A fun but sound grammar book; the examples are thoroughly modern. If you are having basic problems, however, then a simpler text may be better for you.

Halio, Marcia Peoples. (1999). *Writing on the Internet: Finding a voice online*. Fort Worth, TX: Harcourt Brace College Publishers.

This book, based on a course for arts students taking an online course, covers such topics as print versus online writing and how to search for information, find news and support groups, link and work with other students, create a home page, and develop and "publish" a paper. Not an essential for your shelf, but interesting to browse through.

Harbert, E. N., & DiGaetani, J. L. (1984). *Writing for action: A guide for the health care professional*. Homewood, IL: Dow Jones-Irwin.

Out of print, but if you can find it, a terrific book for those of you who will be writing at work. Not really applicable for students. Check libraries and try to borrow a copy if you work in a hospital and have to write reports.

Hodges, John C., Horner, Winifred B., Webb, Suzanne S., Miller, Robert K., Werier, C., & Cohen, Fran. (1999). *Harbrace handbook for Canadians* (5th ed.). Toronto: Harcourt Canada.

A comprehensive review of grammar and punctuation. The last two listed authors are contributors to the Canadian edition, and they have managed to make it a useful Canadian text. Uses the *Gage Canadian dictionary* spellings. Has an excellent chapter on "reading and thinking critically" (pp. 396–418).

Li, Xia, & Crane, Nancy B. (1993). *Electronic style: A guide to citing electronic information*. Westport, CT: Mecklermedia.

A small, expensive book that may be useful for students using many electronic documents in literature reviews and thesis preparation. Needs updating. Mentioned in Chapter 4.

MacLennan, Jennifer. (1995). *Effective business writing* (2nd ed.). Scarborough, ON: Prentice-Hall Canada.

A basic book on letters, memos, reports, and résumés with many examples showing formats and layouts. Also contains useful general comments on ways to develop a clear, concise, complete, and courteous business writing style.

Markman, R. H., Markman, P. T., & Waddell, M. L. (1994). *10 steps in writing the research paper* (5th ed.). Hauppauge, NY: Barron's Educational Series.

Reference used in Chapter 2.

Mascara, Cynthia, Czar, Patricia, & Hebda, Toni. (2001). *Internet resource guide for nurses* (2nd ed.). Upper Saddle River, NJ: Prentice Hall.

An excellent little (106 pages) book that contains, among other things, a long list of World Wide Web sites useful to nurses; unfortunately, these are mostly American and few Canadian resource sites are listed. Because Internet addresses change frequently you need to watch for later editions as well.

Merriam-Webster dictionary of English usage. (1989). Springfield, MA: Merriam-Webster.

This basic reference book on English usage is arranged like a dictionary. In many instances it may tell you more than you wish to know about a subject, but it is perhaps the most useful modern manual on distinctions in usage, although it is decidedly American. If you are an advanced student, you may want it, but a *good* dictionary that explains distinctions in usage will be suitable for most students.

Merriam-Webster's collegiate dictionary (10th ed.). (1998). Springfield, MA: Merriam-Webster.

The latest edition of the dictionary recommended as the spelling standard in the APA (2001) *Manual*. Although there are a number of versions available, this college-level rendering is one of the most complete at a reasonable price.

Miller, Casey, & Swift, Kate. (2001). *The handbook of nonsexist writing: For writers, editors and speakers* (2nd ed.). Lincoln, NE: iUniverse.com.

A new and expanded edition — and you might be surprised at how much you learn by browsing through this! The pages on gender bias in the APA (2001) *Manual* are sufficient for most student writers.

Mirin, Susan Kooperstein. (1981). *The nurse's guide to writing for publication.* Wakefield, MA: Nursing Resources/Concept Development.

Old, but available in many nursing libraries. If you plan to write journal articles, this is one of the best guides there is for nurses — but also apply the SMART principles. It contains excellent information about the organization of articles and gives examples of query letters.

Nemiroff, Greta Hoffman. (1994). *Transitions: Succeeding in college and university.* **Toronto: Harcourt Brace Canada.**

Written for students, this book gives information on anticipating and solving problems that occur during the difficult transition to the postsecondary student lifestyle (e.g., finance, living quarters, study skills, health). Does not deal with writing skills — but with lifestyle challenges (such as living away from home, or making new friends in first year); these often affect your ability to sit down and get started writing.

Northey, Margot, & Timney, Brian. (1995). *Making sense in psychology and the life sciences: A student's guide to writing and style* **(2nd ed.). Toronto: Oxford University Press.**

Out of print, but available in many libraries. Similar to this text, and recommended if you continue to have difficulties with the basic organization of paragraphs and essays. Emphasizes preparation of laboratory reports (e.g., as used in biology or chemistry) and provides excellent examples of grammar and punctuation errors.

Norton, Sarah, & Green, Brian. (2001). *The bare essentials: Form A* **(5th ed.). Toronto: Harcourt Canada.**

An excellent basic grammar text, with lots of exercises — and lots of fun-filled examples. Buy it if you are having serious problems and have the self-discipline to do-it-yourself instead of taking a basic English course.

The pocket Oxford dictionary of current English. **(1978). Oxford, UK: Oxford University Press. (Later editions available)**

Various versions and editions of the *Oxford Dictionaries* are available. As we do not use this dictionary frequently, the version we have is old.

Rockowitz, Murray, Shuttleworth, Dale E., Shukyn, Murray, Brownstein, Samuel C., & Peters, Max. (1998). *How to prepare for the GED high school equivalency exam: Canadian edition* **(3rd ed.). Hauppauge, NY: Barron's Educational Series Inc. (Various later editions, including American editions, available)**

Contains the *best* review of grammar if you are having basic problems (i.e., if you forgot what you learned in grade school). If you are having trouble with the English test required for admission to some colleges or universities, then this is the book for you. As well, any writer would benefit from reviewing the two excellent "Writing Skills" sections. Available in most libraries, including public libraries.

Roman, Kenneth, & Raphaelson, Joel. (1992). *Writing that works: How to improve your memos, letters, reports, speeches, resumes, plans, and other business papers* (2nd ed.). New York: HarperPaperbacks.

A practical little pocketbook that can be helpful with business communications; but think SMART to make it really helpful in health care agencies.

Safire, William. (1990). *Fumblerules: A lighthearted guide to grammar and good usage.* New York: Doubleday.

A fun grammar book — if you already *know* your grammar! — and a wonderful book to browse through to review grammar. (Example from page 79: "Never use a long word when a diminutive one will do.")

Sheridan, Donna R., & Dowdney, Donna L. (1986). *How to write and publish articles in nursing.* New York: Springer.

Old, but texts such as this one no longer seem to be published. You probably will find it in a university or college library. Valuable for students who are good writers and who want to publish while still in the nursing program.

Strunk, William, Jr., & White, E. B. (2000). *The elements of style* (4th ed.). Boston: Allyn and Bacon. (Foreword by Roger Angell)

Strunk and White is the ultimate classic, and professional writers regularly reread this fabulous *small* gem of a book, which reminds them of elementary rules. Everyone recommends it! It was originally written by William Strunk in about 1919, then added to and published in 1959 by E. B. White (author of, among many other more serious books, *Charlotte's Web*); White had been a student of Strunk, and he updated it both in 1959 and then again, with a new chapter, in 1972. Both authors are now dead, but this new edition contains their basic work, plus a few comments related to contemporary writing by White's stepson. Buy this one. Check second-hand stores for the earlier editions to save money, but buy this small, and inexpensive, classic book. Own it, and read it from cover to cover.

Turabian, Kate L. (1996). *A manual for writers of term papers, theses, and dissertations* (6th ed.). Chicago: University of Chicago Press.

A basic style manual written for university students. It used to be the standard style guide for arts courses at universities, and some departments still recommend its use.

Vipond, Douglas. (1996). *Success in psychology: Writing and research for Canadian students.* Toronto: Harcourt Brace Canada.

Somewhat similar to this text, but for students majoring in psychology. It contains an excellent section, "Working the Library," and another on preparing poster presentations if you are asked by an instructor to do this special kind of communication.

Webster's standard American style guide. (1985). Springfield, MA: Merriam-Webster.

A *general* style guide, and an excellent one, although not really applicable to nursing papers. Borrow from a library and browse if you have time.

Woodford, F. Peter. (1999). *How to teach scientific communication.* Bethesda, MD: Council of Science Editors.

If you are going into a master's or doctoral program, you should at least review a copy of this excellent reference tool for graduate students. This is the new edition of *Scientific Writing for Graduate Students: A Manual on the Teaching of Scientific Writing,* written and published in 1986 by the Council of Biology Editors, which has now changed its name to the Council of Science Editors.

Zimmerman, Doris P. (1997). *Robert's rules in plain English.* New York: HarperPerennial.

Many different versions of *Robert's Rules of Order,* first published in 1876 and revised at least 10 times since then, are available. This handy little book is good for general student use; get a 700-page one if you decide to become a parliamentarian. Mentioned in Chapter 6.

Zinnser, William. (1990). *On writing well: An informal guide to writing nonfiction* (4th ed.). New York: Harper Perennial.

A classic book about writing and one recommended in most university English courses.

INDEX